Epilepsy You're Not Alone

Epilepsy You're Not Alone

An Epileptic's View On How To Cope With The Disorder

Written by Stacey Chillemi

Writer's Showcase

San Jose New York Lincoln Shanghai

Writer's Showcase
an imprint of iUniverse, Inc.

For information address:
iUniverse, Inc.
5220 S. 16th St., Suite 200
Lincoln, NE 68512
www.iuniverse.com

ISBN: 0-595-19526-1

Printed in the United States of America

To my husband,
my son Michael
and my
daughter Alexis

CONTENTS

ACKNOWLEDGMENTS

Writing this book was a project that could not possibly have been accomplished by myself. The book was created by the mixture of thoughts, ideas, experiences, and lives who have help change my life. My motivation to write this book began when I walked into a book store and was appalled to find so few books on the topic of epilepsy. It made me even angrier to find that a majority of the books were written by doctors seemly for doctors. The vocabulary and the approach made them difficult for the reader to understand.

At that point, I knew that I wanted to change the way society looked at epileptics, and epileptics looked at themselves. I wanted people to understand what epilepsy is and what it does to people who suffer with the disorder. So I decided to write a book about epilepsy recalling my own and other people's personal experiences with the disorder. I wanted to help other epileptics with this book and educate individuals who knew nothing about epilepsy.

I cannot even begin to express my thanks to all the people who helped me with this book. I first must give appreciation to my husband Michael and my son Mikey and my daughter Alexis, who gave me encouragement to write this book. You stood by my side through all the difficult times I had dealing with epilepsy. To all my family, friends and love ones who have played a big role in my life and has supported all my decisions that I made concerning epilepsy. I would like to express my deepest gratitude to all of you.

I was stunned when I began reading everyone's letters to find how similar we are emotionally about having epilepsy, and how similar our thoughts were about living and coping with epilepsy. We all struggled trying to make our family and loved ones understand how we felt about epilepsy Your letters showed me how I was not alone and that there are many other epileptics battling epilepsy. I also realized through these something I did not recognize before that was that there are many other individuals who have a worse case of the disorder, so there is no reason to pity yourself. You need to get on with life and do something worthy for yourself and others. So my special thanks goes to Adeline A. Napolitano, Melissa Helland, Mary Ellen Reynolds, Ed Schott, Faith Shives, Jerry Griffice, Patrica Otake, Larry Daniel, Darlene McLaughlin, Michael Chupa Jr., Dana Schwartzberg, Debra Ann Knudsen, Donna Letham, Ruth Ann Ray, Vanessa Lovell, Cindy Holsing, Francine Pinkowitz, Betty Brown, Cindy Dailey,Carolyn Bowman, Sherry Kocha. I would like to just thank everyone who has helped me and motivated me to write this book. God bless you all.

INTRODUCTION

Epilepsy has been on this planet as far back as time will take us. According to the Epilepsy Foundation of America, they have quoted some of history's finest to have epilepsy. Not all these are confirmed as having epilepsy, but they state that Alexander the Great had epilepsy (356-323 B.C.), Alfred the Great, West Saxon King and scholar (849-899), Hector Berlioz, French Composer (1803-1869), Julius Caesar (100—44 B.C.), St. Paul the apostle, Socrates the Greek philosopher and mathematician, and Vincent Van Gogh the Dutch painter. Anyone can have epilepsy.

Before we go any further let's ask ourselves the question "what is epilepsy?" Epilepsy is caused by sudden, brief changes in a person's brain activity. When brain cells fail to function properly due to epilepsy, a person's awareness and movements may be altered, perhaps dramatically, for a short period. These sudden physical changes in brain activity are called epileptic seizures.

A person's brain cells usually transmit information to the rest of the body by way of orderly electrochemical signals. These signals are not transmitted randomly; they do not course pell-mell through our nervous system. They are, rather, transmitted selectively, as some messages are inhibited and others allowed to continue on. This selectively prevents "cross talk" or message overload in the body's communication system.

Occasionally, however, a group of brain cells *simultaneously* "fires" or discharges a large number of electrical signals that produce a temporary rise in activity in certain parts of the brain, thus disrupting a person's internal communication system. This is a seizure. A seizure disturbs a person's consciousness, much in the way a lighting storm can disturb the electrical power supply". Each time I have a daytime seizure, I would feel like I put my hand in a socket and was getting electrocuted. The electrical feeling would begin in my feet and travel up my leg through my body. Once the electrical feeling reached my head that would be the moment where I would lose consciousness. The worst part of my seizure is have to feel this electrical current travel through out my entire body. So try closing your eyes for a moment and visualize a lighting storm and how it affects an electrical power supply. This is very much what is happening inside a person's head when he or she is having a seizure. This disruptive overload of brain activity causes the strange body movements, unusual changes in speech, blank stare, and twitching of the eyes (clonic attack extremities) which are symptomatic of epileptic seizures.

A single seizure, bear in mind, does not necessarily signal epilepsy. Epilepsy involves recurrent seizures, varying from one or more a day, to one a month or even as few as one or two year.

Seizures have many causes, epilepsy being only one of them. Having one or two seizures does not mean someone has epilepsy. Non-epileptic seizures can be caused by, among other things, high fevers, and alcohol withdrawal.

Epilepsy affects one to two percent of the United States population. Occurring ten times more frequently than multiple sclerosis and 100 times more frequently than the motornueron disease. Epilepsy affects millions people worldwide, with more than two million people in the United States alone.

Statistics show that one out of twenty people will have at least one seizure associated with epilepsy in his or her life. One out of 200 will ultimately develop full-blown epilepsy. According to the Epilepsy Foundation of America the causes of 70% of all cases of epilepsy are unknown.

Unfortunately, epilepsy is not understood by most people. I am writing this book, therefore, to help people with epilepsy better understand their disorder and also to educate the general public. Many epileptics that I spoke with tell me that they feel their friends, family and doctors don't understand what their going through having to live with epilepsy. It's hard for others to understand the fear you carry inside yourself not knowing when the next seizure is going to occur. How you feel when your having a seizure and how you feel afterwards. Your family, friends and doctors may not completely understand how you feel, but there are other epileptics that understand what you're going through having to live with epilepsy. You're not fighting this disorder all by yourself. There are many other people everyday struggle with the same frightening and bewildering experiences. I, for one, did not fully understand how widespread epilepsy is until I fully researched this book.

When I first started my research, I published an article in EPILEPSY USA—a small, semi—monthly magazine sponsored by the Epilepsy foundation of America. In the article, I encouraged readers to write about their experiences with epilepsy. Many did write and shared some of their deepest feeling about what it feels like to suffer from epilepsy. Needless to say, everyone's story was different, but their feelings about the disorder were strikingly similar. Most said that in a very basic way they were just trying to live as normal a life as possible in spite of actual seizures and their daily fear that a seizure could occur at any time.

Epilepsy affects every aspect of a person's life. The more frequently a seizure occurs, the more profound, needless to say, is the effect. The after-effects of a seizure can be devastating. A seizure leaves you tired, confused and the possibility of enduring some memory loss. Undergoing a seizure may stop you from being able to perform certain tasks because of the risk of a convulsion which could put that person suffering from the attack in a dangerous position. It may cause to be unable to handle certain responsibilities and can even prevent you from participating in some social functions.

The psychological after effect of seizures can make an individual with epilepsy feel they will be restricted from accomplishing the goals they strive for in life—even small goals like driving a car, diving off a diving board, swimming by yourself or even being able to babysit a friend's child. Some people may feel that these goals are not that important, but the people who have the disorder know that they are very important.

One goal that I had was to drive a car. I was able to drive for a couple of years. Once I began to start frequently having seizures my neurologist asked me to stop driving. I used to get very frustrated not being able to drive a car. I am the type of person who likes to depend on myself and not have to rely on others to help me take care of my responsibilities. I felt frustrated and embarrassed to ask other people to drive me to my destinations. It did not matter that they were my family and friends. I felt people were feeling sorry for me and felt some type of obligation to have to drive me to the places I needed to go. I became depressed for a while and I began feeling sorry for myself, until I stopped and said, "enough is enough."

Surprisingly, I was not the only person who was feeling this way. While researching this book, I found that so many people that have this disorder feel so alone. Many people who have written to me have given up their goals and expectations in life. Their attitude about life is very negative. Many people have given up because they feel they have too many limitations and restraints. Countless individuals who suffer from epilepsy think that they can never accomplish their goals and dreams in life, but I am here to tell you that this is not true.

The trick is to learn how to deal with the hopelessness that your experiencing. I strongly believe the first step is to fully accept that you are epileptic. I taught myself to accept that fact and I have learned how to live with the disorder in the most positive way possible. In this book, I talk about how I taught myself to accept me for who I am.

Another important factor is to understand that you are not battling this disorder by yourself. You need to realize that other individuals can relate to you and can empathize with the pain that you are feeling. We all need to be reassured at one point that there are people who understand where we are coming from. These people are wiling to reach out and give you their support. You need to recognize that these people are not going to give you their help unless you ask for it.

It is important that you learn how to live with epilepsy and endure it. Otherwise, you could end up destroying yourself your relationships with people, your friendships, and your family in the end. Everything you do and say affects the people around you.

Eventually if we do not learn how to deal with all these issues, we could end up really destroying ourselves emotionally, physically and spiritually. This does not have to happen if you do not let it. One way to prevent this from happening is to develop a lifestyle that is suitable for your own needs. You need to make sure that it is a lifestyle that is going to make you happy over time. You need to be your own designer, creating pathways to a fulfilling future.

There is a whole world in front of you. This world has millions of opportunities just waiting for you to encounter. It does not matter what age you are. You can achieve anything you put your mind too. For instance, I graduated college with a degree in business and marketing. I have worked in computers and sales for the past three and a half years. I wrote this book and several newspaper articles on the topic of epilepsy. I am happily married with my first baby on the way. My seizures have been well controlled through medicine, exercise and healthy eating habits. I refuse to let epilepsy stop me from getting to the destination I plan on going. The letters in this book share some emotional triumphs of some experiences individuals with epilepsy have endured. They also tell how having epilepsy has affected them physically. Many people who have written to me have shared the methods they used to defeat epilepsy. So there is hope my friends and no need to give up. You will not lose the battle unless you let yourself loose.

This book gives you the materials you need to gain encouragement and strength to overcome having epilepsy and being able to live life to its fullest. In this book, I want to be able to focus on certain topics related to epilepsy that no one has often discussed. One of my main goals in this book is to help others recognize that life has much to offer. Life does not have to cease just because you have epilepsy. As I mentioned earlier, In this book we will be discussing what people go through emotionally when they have epilepsy. We will be going over different ways to help yourself emotionally, physically and spiritually.

The techniques in this book will help you build the inner power to do anything or become anything you want in life. My approaches for dealing with epilepsy will enable you to reform a better direction in your everyday life of living and dealing with your disorder. Most

important, this book shows you that you are not alone. There are people here that understand what your going through and support you. This program will help you build confidence in yourself Once you establish self-assurance, you will start to see your inner strength boost. When one quality improves, all your other attributes will enhance also. This book will give you the tools to learn how to incorporate epilepsy into your life so you can live with the disorder on a positive note. You can make life anything you want if you have positive goals to focus on and if you have a good understanding of how to approach them.

SECTION ONE

LIVING WITH EPILEPSY

Chapter 1

THE EMOTIONAL SCAR OF EPILEPSY

How Others Feel to Have the Disorder

What happens when we have a seizure? We lose control of our body. This is what happens to someone every time a person has a seizure. Such a person has no way to stop the seizures, is unable to stand up, to speak and unable to remember what happened once the seizure is over. Imagine trying to get through life having to live with the constant fear of when and where your next seizure will occur.

Having to cope each day with these unsettled emotions is tough. Emotions such as fear, anxiety, and anger build up inside until you cannot deal with them any longer. Many people with epilepsy feel as though they are alone. They feel they are trying to battle the disorder all by themselves. People who do not have the disorder, ask me "How can epileptics feel they are battling epilepsy alone when they have doctors, family and friends to comfort them". To live with the disorder, one needs to communicate with people who have the same disorder. It gives one the opportunity to open your heart and share your unsettled emotions about how it feels to have epilepsy.

One way of doing this is to subscribe to Epilepsy USA. This is a small newspaper that the Epilepsy Foundation writes. They send the newspaper to you every two months once you become a member. The newspaper informs you about what is going with epilepsy. It has a section where it lists addresses of others with epilepsy that are looking for pen pals. The newspaper also tells you about different events around the states that are constantly going on that you can participate in. For information you can write to the main Epilepsy Foundation in Maryland.

The address is:

4351 Garde City Drive
Landover, MD 20785

If you do not already subscribe to this newspaper than I strongly suggest that you begin too. The newspaper is one way to help give you encouragement, so you can focus on your life and look at epilepsy in a positive way.

This is important because one can easily become depressed focusing on the negative aspects of epilepsy and wallowing in self-pity. This is why support from other individuals who suffer from the same disorder is so important. Understanding what someone with the disorder goes through is difficult, if you don't experience it yourself.

Epileptics from the US and Canada have written the letters in this book. Their stories will help you understand that you are not alone and do not have to battle this disorder all by yourself. Many people with epilepsy struggle just the same as you do, but refuse to let the disorder control them. They have learned to enjoy life by making the best of what God has given them.

After reading these letters your outlook on having epilepsy will begin to change and you will begin to view epilepsy more positively. They will comfort you. Other epileptics understand what you are going through and want to fight this battle by your side.

It amazed me to find that so many of these people who wrote me struggled with similar problems when it came to dealing with epilepsy. The letters in this chapter are from many friends I have made while writing this book, who shared their most deepest intimate thoughts and feelings about living with epilepsy with me. They have also revealed some of their highs and lows.

I hope after reading this chapter, you will realize many other people with epilepsy share the same feelings as you do. I was not the only one struggling to find the miracle drug so one day I could become seizure free. I was not the only one worrying when my next seizure was going to occur. Growing up I always felt that I had to prove I was the same as everyone one else. I should have realized from the beginning that I was no different. There are many people in the world who struggle daily to live a normal life in a society where people can sometimes be very cruel.

I hope these letters will be an inspiration and help you to realize that you are not alone. I hope you enjoy these letters and I hope they will help you as much as they have helped me.

Dear Stacey,

Hi! I received your letter today, and I was glad to get it. It sounds like your taking care of yourself well. It is kind of hard for me to think of babies because I am afraid that something bad would happen to me or the baby or to both of us. You seem healthy. I know the good Lord will take care of you and your baby.

Hopefully, this will cure my fear of having babies, when I see you and your bouncing joy, hand in hand or arm in arm. Depending on how you want to look it. It's great that you can stand on your own two feet, Stacey. Stacey, you have the talent to get other people started, too. Your writing is very powerful. Never forget that.

I am finally able to stand on my own two feet with the medicine Pazil. It is an antidepressant. First, the Epilepsy Foundation is a brilliant place to go for people with epilepsy. They could find out what was wrong with me. I needed to get a sense of responsibility back. I am a more organized person. I get along better with people and even get a lot done in a day.

Praises are to God. I lost 49 lbs., and my heaviest was 205 lbs. Now I am down to 156, and I would like to get down to 130-135 lbs. The Neurontin I am taking is 1200 mg. Last week I had many seizures. I went to my doctor Monday. My doctor thought it was the bad news I received the previous Tuesday. I applied for a full-time job at a light factory. It would have been a great job for me, unfortunately, they wrote me a letter stating that they filled the position. So I have to try harder next time. I know that someone out there has to give me a job. I have really come a long way. My husband and I could go over to my friend's house and spend the day with her, then we took her to group at the Epilepsy Foundation. There was a movie that night.

Take Care and God Bless,
Have a Great Day!!!!

I think this lovely lady who has epilepsy was able to turn her life around with the help of others. The Epilepsy Foundation helped her move on with her life. She was able to communicate with other epileptics through the Epilepsy Foundation. The epileptics she met through the foundation filled her heart with hope and happiness. The foundation made living with epilepsy much easier.

Dear Stacey,

Hello. How's things going? I am doing fine here in Grove City. Thank you for your uplifting letter and your article. You seem like a kind, loving person yourself. I come from a family of loving people, we learned young in life to take care of ourselves and help each other. My parents not only taught, but showed the way.

I am in the middle of eight brothers and sisters (five brothers and three sisters). I was born in 1953. I am right in the middle. My oldest sister died in 1963, she had a rare disorder that caused her major organs to age rapidly. My brother and I had neumatic fever. I was five at the time. I learned how precious life is and how easily it can be taken away.

We were poor. Although my father had a good job, there were eight kids. We learned to depend on each other and to trust each other. Oh, we had our misunderstandings with each other. My oldest brother is one of my best friends in the world.

Well, so much for my family history. By the way I am the second oldest of the boys. All of my sisters were older. In 1989, I was walking home from work (about 1 mile), the temperature outside was thirty. The first day of winter.

I arrived at my trailer, and I took my glove off my left hand. The next thing I know a cop (a good friend) was calling out to me, he was aware of my seizures. My hands were so cold, even the one with the glove on it. I was shivering.

Suddenly a squad came into the lot and over to me. I have never been that cold before. I had fallen from my seizures (That is usual; I fall backwards and to the left a little when I have a seizure). Before I regained my awareness I got up and started walking, unaware of what was happening (also, usual). I walked into the trailer hit my head and passed out. I was lying in the snow and as I said, it was 30 degrees for a half hour or forty-five minutes.

They got me on the stretcher and started putting hot water bottles around me. They took my temperature. I heard one person say "Going into hyperthermia. His is below critical. The next day I woke up in a hospital. The knuckle in my left hand (the one unclosed) was aching badly. Soon after the doctor came into the room with bad news and good news to tell me. Oh no! I thought. He said, "First the bad news: you have first degree frost bite." I braced myself for the next sentence. "The good news: you get to keep your fingers." I was so happy and relieved that tears were running down my face. First degree frost bite is the mildest form of a frost bite.

Now, it is still something I have to deal with. Yet I will exchange it for my fingers any time! I really do not like to tell these stories and do not want people to feel sorrow or pity for me. Hey, I have had seizures for going on a quarter of a century. I take care of myself. I am very independent. For sure I do not suffer as much as many other people with epilepsy. I am truly one of the lucky ones. I have had thousands of seizures over the years and I am here telling you about some. How many can say they never lost the ability to take care of themselves?

Keep up the faith and live the good life.

P.S. My dad had a saying about life; nobody gets out of this alive. He is right, we live life as full as we can. **One Day at A Time!**

I learned from this letter that support from others can be very crucial in overcoming any obstacle from epilepsy that comes our way. Inner strength is something we need to overcome epilepsy. And you can develop inner strength through support and love from the people who mean the most to us in life and that can understand what we're going through. You need to take in consideration that inner strength does not happen overnight, so be patient and live life "One Day at A Time!"

Dear Stacey,

Hi, I am forty-nine years old. When I first started having seizures, I had no aura, so I did not know when these seizures were about to happen. People were horrified when I had a seizure. They scattered as if they thought it was contagious. They never realized how much hurt and fear inside me was beyond their knowledge! When one of these seizures hit me there was nothing I could do, but go through it. Not many people understand that even today! Sometimes when I am having a seizure I can feel the blood because my head would hit the ground so hard like a 10-pound sledge hammer in full swing!

Stacey, the only way to get better is by God and your medicine in that order. You need to put your faith first. I believe if it were not for God that I would not be writing this letter today. I would be dead! I also believe that you need to think positively in this life. You should always look forward and never look backwards, tomorrow is another day.

I am fine for right now. I had two seizures in the chiropractor's office and four coming home, which knocked me down each time. Nevertheless, being "mule-headed" I got right back up! Until the last one knocked a hole in my elbow and I had to get a couple of stitches. I had to take a ride in the ambulance, which I really did not want to do.

I have had seizures for twenty-nine years. The medicine that I take is Depakene (Valporic Acid), Neurontin and Dilantin. Neurontin has been the best medicine that I ever took.

I believe this epileptic did not let epilepsy control his life. He used God to help him develop his inner strength and to look at his life in a positive way. In order to develop inner strength. You need to have a clear mind so you can make productive goals for your life. You need to reach out for help. You cannot win this fight with epilepsy by yourself.

Dear Stacey,

Congratulations on your pregnancy! I am so happy for you; you must be thrilled! I was not on any medications during my two pregnancies, only because I did not know that I was having seizures, I never dreamed that I had epilepsy. My seizures started the month I turned twenty-six years' old. (July 1980), when I first became pregnant with my first child, (my daughter). During both my pregnancies I felt great, I worked all the time and I was very happy. The only "black cloud," were these awful "spells," that I was having. I did not know that I was having seizures until one year after my second child, (my son), five years after my first "spell!"

They diagnosed me with simple-partial seizures, which eventually worsen to complex- partial seizures. Twice I suffered status-epileptics resulting in generalized seizures, which required hospitalization.

I am still in school (Henry Ford Community College, Dearborn, Michigan. Last semester I had two (kind of) tough classes, but I loved them. Pathophysiology and Pharmacology and I was proud of my grades, B&A-, respectively. This semester I have only one class, Medical Computer Information Systems, but I am finding this one class more difficult than last semester's two classes combined.

I am hoping to take a spring and summer class. I have switched from medical transcription (a certificate), to Medical Information Technology (an associate's degree). So I will have a better degree!

Take care, God Bless,

I believe this epileptic did not let epilepsy control her. She was blessed with two healthy children and is working on her college degree. You don't have to stop living just because you have epilepsy. She focused on her goals and looked positively at life. This is what you need to do.

Dear Stacey,

I am twenty-nine years old. I have had seizures for almost ten years now. My general experience with epilepsy has been pretty interesting. When I first had the seizures, my family was completely shocked, including my grandmother who has since past away. Nobody ever knew what caused me to have the seizures and they still do not know the reason what caused me to have the seizures. There were tons of tests done and nothing came out of it. My experience with epilepsy was a painful one. My seizures came about very suddenly. At first the neurologist put me on Dilantin. Bad move. Why? Because it caused my gums to swell like balloons. That required some surgery. Everyone in my family thought I would die of these seizures. After each one, I had become very light headed for a brief period.

When I was working, my co-workers were very supportive of me. The same holds true for both my family and friends. When my grandmother was alive at the time that I had the first seizures, she was extremely supportive of me. She even came to the hospital to see how I was doing. She was like that until about two months before she passed away. This was three years ago. After that her health failed rapidly. Anytime I did not feel too good after having the seizures, all I had to do was call her. She would make me feel much stronger. I feel that living with epilepsy is easy!! With the combination of both my family and friends, and the fact that I take my medication religiously on time every day, my life is extremely easy! My family and friends continue to support me while I have epilepsy. You definitely have to think positively and forget the past! Think about your future!

I like bike riding, miniature golf, walking and flea markets, garage sales, archery and of course, shopping! I also collect Sylvester the cat stuff. My collection is pretty big and it continues to grow. I am a 70's music fan, and love music from the 80's and 90's as well. I am also an Elvis fan, a Beatles fan, and a U2 fanatic.

I think this young lady used support from her family and friends to help her gain a sense of inner strength. She did not fall into depression because she focused on her goals and interests. She also looked at life positively by not focusing on her past. She focused on the good things to happen in her future.

Dear Stacey,

I often read the letters in Epilepsy USA, so I have found yours quite interesting. I found growing up what they finally diagnosed as psychomotor epilepsy rather than petite-mal.

I had removal of 2/3 of the right temporal lobe and graduated in 1958. Try explaining that to those many people who through the years looked at me as though (and thought) the devil possessed me or else I was a witch! People kept children in some cases from playing with me.

I could not really understand what was happening to me or why. It was not something that we discussed outside the family either.

In fact, to the day she died last year, my mother was horrified that I should tell my friends I had epilepsy! After all what would her friends think.

I went off to college to major in agriculture. I found out that due to surgery my seizures were less. Nevertheless, the people with whom I was in contact accepted my epilepsy and my social life was great.

I'm convinced students away for college drop the fear of their parents! Bosses, friends and, of course, my husband accept my epilepsy-that's the way it has gone.

Dear Stacey,

I believe this epileptic had difficultly growing up with epilepsy because not until recently was epilepsy brought out into the open. Many people did not know what seizures were and when they saw someone go into a convulsion they did not know to react. Epileptics were looked at strangely and were singled out. This strong young lady did not let her past effect her. She went on with her life and got a college degree. She met friends who accepted her epilepsy. She got married and created a family for herself. She reached out for help through medical attention and the magazine Epilepsy USA.

Dear Stacey,

I have simple partial seizures. Sometimes they are borderline complex partial. Medication has not totally controlled my seizures and I am not a candidate for epilepsy surgery. My medication controls my seizures from fifty to sixty seizures a day to seven to twelve a day I had my first seizure at age forty-two. I am now age forty-seven. The doctors do not know why my seizures began. I have had many tests, but no answers. I still hope one day new research will produce a new medicine that will give me freedom from seizures.

I face the challenge of dealing with my epilepsy in many ways. Number one is through prayer. Secondly, I use every chance to educate someone about the subject of epilepsy or seizures. I often find out that many people are surprised that I do not fall onto the floor or violently shake when I have a seizure. They are not aware that there is more than one type of epilepsy. They wrote me once up in a newspaper article for our local paper and were featured in an article about epilepsy for Women's Day magazine. Epilepsy still unfortunately, has many stigmas and until we can talk about it freely and educate the public many those stigmas will remain. A doctor or counselor can talk about it all day. You and I are the people who live with it and should explain to the public like what it really feels like.

I believe this epileptic has also realized that epilepsy is beginning to come out into the open, but there's still a lot of work to be done in educating the public on epilepsy. When I read this letter I felt very proud of her because she used what she had to help others. She reached out so others could understand what the disorder is. By following her goals and dreams she was able to pursue her life and not let epilepsy stand in her way.

Dear Stacey,

My seizures began around my 25th birthday. I had just become pregnant with my first child, (I have two children, my daughter Candice, sixteen years. old, and my son Chad, thirteen year's old. I have continued to work throughout and have raised my children, while I was living and dealing with epilepsy. My seizures were simple and partial. During my years with epilepsy I have had three generalized (Grand-Mal) seizures, one of those times resulted in an episode of status-epileptics, which I am sure you are aware can be life-threatening without hospitalization. Along with epilepsy, they diagnosed and treated me for panic attack disorder. I have my own theory about the connection between seizures and panic attacks. Though I hated what the seizures did to me (and my family) and the ways they made me feel, I was not afraid of them. I still experience a form of panic attack, but the logical reasoning behind them is that it happens when I am subjected to large crowds of people (I feel suffocated). This type of anxiety is totally different (and feels different) from what I had when I was having seizures. (They worsened with my cycle and my pregnancies. Being a woman you are probably very aware of the effect hormones can play on seizures.

I have a recent pen-pal that experiences the same anxiety with her seizure disorder that I did. At the time of my surgery I was thirty-eight years old. My children were eight and eleven years old. They had a lot to deal with. I am forty-three yrs. old (and proud of it), and last year, after being out of school for twenty-four years, I went to college! I love it! I just turned forty-three on July 3rd and my son (who has the same birthday, turned thirteen! I have two teenagers! Am I nuts?!, Oh yes, I am going for my certificate in Medical Transcription. Did I mention that I had continued to work, and had worked (starting after high-school), for physicians, doing their billing and typing their narrative reports? They retired in 1994, and I went on to work for a pharmacist.

I prayed for, and received the courage to go through with the surgery and to be able to reassure my family, as they were wheeling me into the operating room. Yes, I would do it again, you bet. During the almost five years since my surgery I have had only one seizure and that was when I was off all medicines, and had been for nine months. So I am back on my medicines seizure—free again. I take only Dilantin 1OOmg for the seizure-control. Two in the morning and two at bedtime.

Epilepsy? I am not sick, are you? Of course not. We are nice people that have lived with epilepsy. I suppose people are afraid are afraid of the disorder. I did not have fits. I had seizures. The only fits I had, have been when

I have been mad about something, I have been known to have a temper or when one Doctor (Intern, I think) asked me about my "fits."

I believe this epileptic has had a lot to deal with, but through the help of prayer and three healthy children, she was able to receive the support and love she needed to go on with her life. She continued working. She developed productive goals that would make her feel good about herself. She didn't use epilepsy as a crutch. She went on with her life.

Dear Stacey,

Hi! I am twenty-five years old. I am married and have two children. I have a six-year-old named David Cody and a one and a half-year-old girl named Morgan Elizabeth.

David had been sick for a couple of days with a cold. I remember we had a couple of feet of snow that night in January. Two of my girlfriends were visiting and we were all sitting around talking. My husband was holding David over his shoulder. I just happened to glance over at David and his eyes were rolled up in his head. I screamed to my husband, "there is something wrong with David!" At that point his whole body limbed like a rag doll. I lay him down on the floor to see if he were breathing. I could not see his chest moving, so I started to give him CPR. I knew nothing about the seizures at the time. I remember then picking David up in my arms and his little body just laying there limp. I thought he was dead!

The ambulance got there finally and rushed him to Union Hospital, in Maryland. A little while after we got to the hospital; we found out that he had a Febrile seizure. These are quite common for children his age I was glad to hear that! During the next two years he had three more Febrile seizures, which was not too bad.

A couple months after he turned three years old, he started having seizures for no reason. The first time it happened, we rushed him to at Dupont Children's Hospital in Delaware. David had already had two at home then while the doctor was checking him out, he had another one so the doctor gave him Tegretol Rectally. They kept David in the hospital for about four days to make sure his seizures were under control. It was a very scary time for us.

For the next year he did well and his neurologist saw him every three months. After about a year, he started having them again, so they increased his dosage again to four tsp. a day. This went on until he was on six tsp. a day and he started to get into the toxic range to the point where he was totally zoned out, tired. He lost interest in almost everything and could not function.

Preschool was horrible. Even after being on six tsp. a day he was still having seizures, so his doctor put him on Depakote. The doctor weaned him off the Tegretol. At this point we were very frustrated. We felt like all we could do, was sit back and watch him suffer from the side effects of the medications he was taking. At five years old, my son's mentality was delayed. At birth they found that David's corpus callosum was thinner then a normal child's.

The corpus callosum is one of the most striking features of the brain. Its bilateralism, or organization into the largely symmetric left and right cerebral hemispheres. Each hemisphere is independently capable of processing and storing information. In humans and other mammals the corpus callosum is the main pathway of interhemispheric communication. The callosum is the largest fiber tract in the human brain, containing more than 200 million nerve fibers (axons).

It's critical role was demonstrated by Ronald Myers and Roger Sperry in the 1950s, when they showed (in cats) that information reaching one half of the brain was unavailable to the other half when the callosum was absent.

In the 1960s in Sperry's laboratory, Joseph Bogen and Peter Vogel cut the callosum in a group of epileptic human patients in an effort to control their otherwise unmanageable seizures. The psychological follow-up of the patients by Michael Gazzaniga, Sperry, and Bogen confirmed the earlier animal studies. Studies of the left and right hemispheres in human beings have revealed the psychological uniqueness of the separate hemispheres.

The left hemisphere is normally dominant for language functions. The right one seems to be better equipped for handling spatial and other nonverbal relations. Such observations have led to theories suggesting hemispheric specialization through evolution. For example, investigators such as Gazzaniga and Joseph LeDoux suggest that human hemispheric differences can be accounted for in terms of the evolutionary acquisition of language by one hemisphere. The other hemisphere continues to process information essentially as it did in prehumans. The superior performance of the right hemisphere on certain nonverbal tests would then be attributable to the sacrifice of nonverbal processing efficiency by the left hemisphere because of having acquired language.

Research shows that double consciousness exists in split-brain patients. Perhaps a fully integrated consciousness does not develop until a child is several years old. Research shows that the fibers of the corpus callosum do not begin to mature until one year after birth, and that the process continues until the age of ten or older. The corpus callosum has also been found to be about 11% larger in left-handed and ambidextrous than in right-handed people.

David also had other problems with his reflex, he had six toes on each foot. Three toes on each foot are webbed together and his two middle fingers on his left hand were also webbed together. He had surgery on his fingers in January, to separate them. It was very successful. David's been going to a school that specializes in kids with special needs. He has been going there since he was ten months old. David's fine and gross motor skills are at a four-year old level. His speech is at a three-year-old level.

At that point in my son's life, between the seizures and the medications, I started to look for alternatives to David's problem. I was not quite satisfied with what the doctors had to offer my son. It seemed like it all revolved around drugs and that was the extent of it. So, I went to one of my friend's nutritionist, who firmly believes in the benefit of the Shaklee supplements. These supplements are diet containing generous amounts of fresh vegetables, fruits, dairy products, and meat which assures an adequate intake of vitamins and minerals, which my son had been lacking all along. So I sat and talked with her about all my concerns for David. She got very excited. She said, "Marybeth, if you really get serious about rebuilding your son's state of health, this means making sure he gets his food supplements every day and change some of the things he eats in his diet."

Naturally I went home very excited. I started him on supplements right away and got rid of all my household cleaners and replaced them with Shaklee Cleaners, which are all biodegradable and nonchemical. For the first thirty days, my sons' body went through a cleansing, because when you introduce organic foods and all those nutrients and minerals; the body will automatically eliminate toxins and start to heal. After about thirty to thirty-five days, boy, did I start to see drastic changes with David. On of the most vivid things was he had lots of energy, and he was not pale and washed out anymore. His cheeks became rosy, and started to talk more and he was showing interest again in doing everyday things like going to the playground, swimming, and socializing with other kids. There was a major improvement in his health. He was always sick with something from the time he was one to five years old and taking antibiotics at least once a month. They hospitalized him at least twice a year with pneumonia or bronchitis. He was then of course having seizures. He was a very sick child!

It has been nine months since he has been on the Shaklee diet and has only been to the doctor for an ear infection once. At David's school his teachers were saying what an improvement David is making. They said that he stopped taking naps in class and his attention span was better. His concentration and balance showed major improvement! In as little as two months, my child went from being a very sickly, unhappy, tired and zoned out kid to being a child with energy. He is very healthy, he is alert and he has not had a seizure in over a year. He is on Depakote and we are still weaning him off the Tegretol. It is a very slow process. Let me tell you what we are currently giving David to supplement his diet:

EACH DAY

Two tsp. a day of liquid tea (Panathonic Acid Biotin Riboxlauch Niacin vitamins A, D, B, B's, Iron)
two glasses of Soy protein (very important in brain function and energy)
Six EPA capsules (fish oil)
6 Lecithin Capsules (helps nervous system and brain function)
2 Formula I capsule (mixture of antioxidenenls and B's that help boost the Zinc selenium immune system vitamin C)
4 GLA (essential fatty acid)
Six chewable C
2 Bett Tacarotene (builds immune system and fights against cancer)
Fiber Waters chewable-vitamin E 200 IU (The body's natural broom. it keeps the toxin out of the body.)
This is what I give him every day. I just poke a hole in the capsules and squeeze them into the liquid tea and he drinks it down. The reason that I chose to give the Shaklee supplements to my son is because I know that they are safe. Shaklee is the only company that does clinical studies and scientific research on their product before they market them. So when I give Shaklee to David I know that he is getting the best out there!

I truly believe that they introduced me to Shaklee for a reason. It was definitely a work of God! I would really hate to think of the shape my son would be in now without the Shaklee products.

I feel like I have a mission here. Think about all the people out there stricken with epilepsy that not only have to deal with the seizures, but have to deal with the side effects of the drugs!

This was a challenge, but I believe that God is in control of everything that happens in peoples lives. In know that my David is in Gods hands and God will take care of him better than anyone else!

God does everything for a reason, we just have to have faith. We just have to have faith that there is a reason behind everything God does. When were going through bad times with David. I could have blamed

God, and said, "Why does this have to happen to our child?" Yet through it all I have learned how to be thankful for the little things. It has made me a stronger person and has made my husband and I a lot closer and stronger together. Greatest of all, I feel that now I can be of great benefit to other parents who have children suffering from epilepsy.

I really believe that diet supplements and getting rid of chemicals in the home is vital to people suffering from epilepsy. David has shown amazing results!

I think everything happens for a reason. David's parents can use this experience to help others. David's parents used their faith in God to help them through this tough period in their lives. They didn't give up hope and they used their inner strength to search a for solution to help their son's seizure disorder. Diet supplements may not help everyone, but in this case it was very helpful in David's situation.

Dear Stacey,

I am forty-four years old, and my first known seizure was at the age of twenty. At age five years, I had a high fever that caused convulsions. My older brother told me when he saw me have my first seizure that looked like when I was five years old and had convulsions. He was nine years old at the time.

I work at a grocery store. I do not drive and live alone. So I walk about 95% of the time I do not want to drive. I worry about hurting or even killing somebody else.

On February 3, 1994, I went to my neurologist. I was using a new anti—convulsion medicine called Felbatol. I got a bad side effect from the medication so the doctor put me back on Tegretol. Later he added Neurontin to try to help control the seizures better.

During the change over I had a seizure while walking to work. It was cold and snowing (I fall to the left slightly, then backwards with my seizures) I fell and landed in the snow and slid into the street under a car.

When I have seizures, I do not become mentally aware until five to ten minutes afterwards. I never remember any of my seizures. I pulled myself from under the car and kept going to work I heard people yelling for me to stay, they were asking " Is your head all right? " I did not understand because I was still dazed from the seizure. About two or three minutes later a policeman pulls over to the curb and walks over to me. He said, "Are you OK?" I said, "yes". He said, "Don't you know where you were, being dragged down the street by a car? I said, "A car?" "He said, "You did not know it, did you?" I said, "No sir." I did know my hip area was starting to hurt and I felt I was walking funny. The police officer said, "Well an ambulance is on the way." I said, "I don't have time, I have to get to work before 9:00 p.m.. I also have to pick up my medicine before the pharmacy closes."

By the time we were through the squad car arrived. They said, "lie on this, so we can take you to the hospital." I said, "No thanks," and went on to work. I lasted about a half hour. Sitting, standing, and laying down; nothing would ease my pain.

While I was trying to work, the gentleman who was driving the car noticed me. He was going to the store. He said, "Excuse me, sir." I said, "Yes sir." He said, he was driving the car that took me down the street. My heart ached for him, I was stunned!

I said, "Please forgive me, but I just had one of my seizures. Don't worry, I think we both should feel lucky that it is just my hip and you did not run me over. "I feel bad when others are involved this way. It does not seem fair. This person was not doing anything wrong. We need to consider others who, by being in the wrong place at the wrong time are feeling, caring people and need help too.

Well, after about half an hour of work, I asked one of my coworkers to call a squad car. They did and I went to get medical attention. To this day, I still feel bad for the driver. My area between my waist and knees are a problem. Nevertheless, I still walk 95% of the time and work full time. I take no pain killers. I just go on.

I told you about my high fever, but that is not the source of the seizures (or not the main source). Sometime between 1953 and 1962 I had a hit on the head above the right eye; so hard that the retina right ripped and partially detached from the optic nerve. This may be one of the causes of my epilepsy. My right frontal lobe is where my seizure's starts. When the doctors look in my right eye they said they could do nothing because the detachment was not fresh enough. I started to fall on the left side first. I knew this because its my left hip that's hurt from the falls 98% or more of the time. It was not until 1973 my first known seizure occurred.

My neurologist told me that I 'm not a candidate for surgery. It was not worth the risk because my seizures are under good control with medicine. I dropped from hundreds of seizures a year to two or three dozen. So I am close to seizure-free. I also have auras'. My auras are really scary, the taste in my mouth is terrible and my tummy feels like I have gas in it. I get goose bumps from head to my toes with the exemption of the very top of my head.

I think epilepsy has put quite a few obstacles in this gentleman's life, but as you can see he has not let having epilepsy get him down. He has focused on the positive aspects of his life and this has given him the strength that he needs to go on with his life. He has accepted that he has epilepsy and he knows epilepsy is a part of his life. This is why he is able to cope with his epilepsy.

Dear Stacey,

I am forty-five years old. I am presently living with my parents since my dad is in a wheelchair. My dad has diabetes. I help take care of him. I have petite-mal seizures and have been having seizures since I was sixteen months old. I have tried all kinds of medications, but none seem to work. However, I am now trying the new drug called Topamax. I usually have a few seizures at the time of my menstrual period.

My parents and I have gone to support group meetings. They discuss new medicines and ways to control seizures. I enjoy the support group meetings and can meet other people who also have seizures.

I believe support group meeting are beneficial people who have epilepsy in their families. Many people find them informative and comforting.

Stacey,

The weather has been perfect for me to get out and get busy. The only downside is that I overdo the work or play and finds me with a head that feels like a sparkler on the fourth of July. I noticed three things you said in your last letter that I can relate to:

1. Those without seizures do not understand completely. I use to tell my doctors, "I wish you could live one month with my symptoms

Maybe then you be more sympathetic." You're right! Family and friends listen, but they do not really understand! Only another person with the problem can fully understand what we go through. That is my big problem. People think I should be the "superman" I used to be. I cannot. They do not understand why. I try to keep going, but I am destroying my body. I have fallen so often during the last few years, it is a wonder I can still walk. I used to like to stay on the road, and do weekend trips. I know now, a 50-mile trip will put me in bed for a day or two. I do not like my brain feeling like oatmeal, sparking, or feeling like it's spinning in six different directions, in addition to all the other symptoms. I do not like feeling bad, so I am avoiding things that hurt me. People do not understand.

2. You mention about what is "Normal." I have had doctors ask me if I feel normal after taking a different medication. I replied, "What is normal?" "What is normal for you surely is not normal for me." Stacey, I thought I was normal for twenty-eight years. You know why you have seizures, and I don't. I guess the only difference is that you are not in the dark and you knew you had a problem since youth.

3. Mind over matter…when I was much younger and into the martial arts, I learned a great deal about mind over matter. I could direct pain out of my body by focusing on something else. I used to be able to obtain an 8-hour sleep in five minutes. (Sounds goofy, but it works.) I know all about mind over matter, but when the mind does not function right, you cannot control anything. When my brain shorts out, I am done. No control, I am at the mercy of what happens next. I have tried to control the seizures. I have not been able to, so far, any more

than the medication controls it. I will not give up. I still do more than I should, but that is me. I never give up. I do not like having no control of my thoughts. Sometimes I have no thoughts at all. I also experience temporarily and short term memory loss. This started five to seven years ago. This is not good either.

I feel like you have a good handle on life. You make the most out of life that you can. I wasted too many years, trying to deny my problem, then being depressed. I'm now trying to figure what the future holds for me.

I am stubborn, I will not give up and I keep Jesus in my heart. It did not matter how tough it was; when my life did a one hundred and eighty degree turn, he was the only one who understood. He was the only one that was there when I needed someone the most.

I believe this epileptic is still struggling with epilepsy, but with the help of religion and by reaching out to other epileptics she has begun to see the brighter side of life. She has opened her heart and her mind and has begun to listen to what other epileptics have to say. She realizes that she is not the only one who feels the way she does.

Dear Stacey,

I am a 66-year-young female. I was first diagnosed to have some form of epilepsy at the age of forty-seven. This was very shocking to me.

I saw a neurologist who then diagnosed me as having psychomotor seizures or complex partial seizures. I have been on many medications; Dilantin, Phenobarbital, Mysolin, just to name a few and have seen many neurologists. I went through all the side effects and the medication did not help.

I have been on Tegretol for seven years and thank God I do not have any side effects. It seems to agree with me, although my seizures are not under complete control. Of course I do not know what it's doing to my inside. Time alone will tell. I really do not like changing medications, because of all the side effects.

I have to agree with you when you say friends and family members assume that whenever something is happening to you it is because of the epilepsy. It drives me crazy. They immediately say, "Did you take your medicine?"

When they told me originally I was epileptic I cried for days. My family could not understand why it was so upsetting to me. When I look back, I can only say that I was ignorant about epilepsy. I thought of this as a horrible curse coming over me and did not understand that there were all types of seizures. My family and friends accepted me for who I was and never let it interfere with our relationship. They were and still are very caring.

After a long while, I finally accepted that I am epileptic and live as normal a life as I can. Yet I realize that there is nothing I can do to change that, so I do not think about it anymore. I worked in the telephone company for thirty-seven years before retiring in 1985. The last six years were difficult. I could not drive anymore and it was tiring getting back and forth to work. Again, my friends came through most of the time.

I was driving for years. I had a motor vehicle accident in 1979 and hit a police car! I did not wait for my license to be taken away; I gave it up myself. Years later I began to drive again. I had a second accident after having a year free of seizures in 1983. This convinced me that I would never drive again. It is very discouraging at times because I live alone. I use to feel sorry for myself, but that is all over now. My friends, family and neighbors help with the transportation. I also use public transportation, when necessary.

Before they diagnosed me with seizures I always remember feeling very strange on and off, but it was my stomach that bothered me or my intestines. Whenever I would tell the doctor he would say, "It is your nerves." Don't you love it?, Always your nerves. Nevertheless, my mother would always look at me and say, "Are you having a problem with your stomach?" Because she said, I always looked a little strange for just a few seconds. This went on for years. My sister said, I was being very rude and just ignoring people.

I do not know when I am getting a seizure and I do not know that I have had one; unless they tell me. They last anywhere from thirty seconds to two or three minutes. I get very tired after having one. I sometimes get up and walk around or just stare. I do not feel sick, just tired. I live a normal life and my friends are aware of my problem, so I'm not afraid to get involved in projects etc.

When they diagnosed me, I was married, but my husband could not accept the fact that I was epileptic so we went our separate ways. I have been alone since 1981. As much as I have accepted the fact that I cannot drive again, it is the only thing that really frustrates me. I love to drive.

I find myself at times feeling very angry because the medicines could not get my seizures under control. I read and talk to many people who have different types of epilepsy and they are under complete control. Most of them are grand-mal, which is a lot worse than mine.

I often wonder why we have so many organizations and celebrities who donate time and money to help find a cure for AIDS, but it seems people have forgotten epileptics. I wonder how others feel about this?

I think there many issues in this letter that I can relate to personally and I'm sure others can too. I have learned from this letter that many individuals do not realize how lucky they are until certain things become impossible for them due to epilepsy. I didn't realize how lucky I was to be able to drive until I had to give up my license because of my seizures. Luckily, there were no major injuries due to the car accident she was involved in. It's better not to drive at all if you are going to put your life or others at risk. When my license was taken away I had to look for other ways of transportation. But the way to deal with this problem is to accept that you have epilepsy and include it into to your life. You cannot put yourself in denial. You must accept your epilepsy and be grateful for what God has given you. In our world full of billions of people, I guarantee there is someone out there worse off then we are. Also, this letter teaches us that because so many people are not educated on epilepsy people tend to think that every time you may not feel well it is because of your epilepsy. This can be frustrating to someone with epilepsy. This is why we all should take time out from our daily schedule to try to help others understand epilepsy. And last but not least remember that if anyone in our lives does not want to accept us for who we are then they do not deserve to have us in their lives.

Dear Stacey,

My husband and I have a newspaper route. It is seven days a week. It makes me feel good about myself. My old self is back! My friend gave me her support. That really did a great job for my self-esteem. Now I feel like I can CONQUER THE WORLD!

I am on Neurontin too for my epilepsy. I see circles at times and I did have a seizure or two. I called my doctor, and he made me increase the Neurontin. That darn epilepsy will always be in my life. Nevertheless, I cannot harp on this. I feel too good about myself.

God Bless,

I believe epilepsy can lower your self-esteem if you let it. This is why you must get out into the world and do things that make you feel good and proud of yourself. Remember in order to help the people around you that you care about, you must first help yourself.

Dear Stacey,

Busy, Busy, Busy! I am trying to find a little time for myself. My daughter is tracking scholarship information and I am working on college financial aid for her. My husband can always find oodles of things for me to do for him. So naturally with the holidays and shopping on everyone schedule. I am bonkers since I cannot drive now. You should see me walking the stress off. I exercise like a "wild woman!"

Loved your article. How inspiring! I have shared it with some people I know will appreciate it and benefit from it. You are now one of my heroes! I wish more people would share their experiences. We need to know how others have felt the same feelings. We have and you know others need to read about it too.

I believe this letters shows the importance of reaching out to others and how it can help change the lives of others who have epilepsy.

Dear Stacey,

I went to Riverside, California. To meet the love of my life. After traveling thirty-six hours on the bus, it was love at first sight for me. We had such a nice time together in California. I really did like it there. Nothing else mattered.

I don't think that I have ever worked as hard in my whole life as I did to get to California. Then something came over this bachelor. The wind was light. It was blowing through the palm trees and the smell of different flowers was in the air. As I turned to her and asked her "Will you marry me?" The look that came over her face was one of great joy. She said, "Well-let me think about it O.K.?" I thought to myself, she will give me a week or so at least to discuss it with her mother. However, I was wrong. She turned to me and said, "Yes." I almost fell like a big oak tree. She asked me if I were all right. I told her yes, just a little "all shook up."

We did not have an engagement ring. So she looked through her jewelry box and found this old ring, which we went and had polished. This ring was so pretty that neither one of us believed it. It was a ruby with pink flowers on all four sides. Now after forty-nine years I finally bit the bullet.

After we had such a great time then, bad luck hits. At 12:03 p.m. The following morning I went to the rest room and afterwards a second later I was thrown against a wall. Somehow I had suffered a bad injury to my right foot. I elevated my foot and then went into several other continuous seizures. When I could get some medicine that my fiancee administered, the seizures than stopped. At six o'clock the next morning I was looking at my foot and I knew that I had to go to the hospital.

The doctor at the hospital told me that I just had a bad sprain and put a splint on the foot. It was tight though; after riding a bus for thirty-six hours, my fiancee and I finally got home and then, we went to the ER. This time they threw away and replaced the splint with a new splint that would allow for the swelling. After taking X-rays, the next morning, I went to my doctor. The doctor told me That I had torn ligaments and had a fractured ankle. The doctor put a fiberglass cast on my right foot up to my calf muscle.

My family likes my fiancee very much, and her friends liked me. I do think that this all means that I have found my partner for life. Epilepsy wise, I've been having five to eight seizures a month, but I am built tough. I hope! Stacey, everyone has their ups and downs, because we are all human. I'm really proud of you for getting off that medicine. I had always had faith in you as a friend and am always your "cheerleader." It will come to pass, if you believe in the Lord and let him show you the way. Trust me, I had a rough trail, but without the Lord I would have had never made it. The words "give up" are not words as they are thought. One must think positively when preparing to face the black knight called epilepsy. Because when you look at epilepsy negatively it will end up controlling your life.

I believe this epileptic's letter is very inspiring. He show's that you can have a happy life living with epilepsy. He is able to live a productive and happy life because he does not look at his disorder negatively.

Dear Stacey,

Hi! How are you? I am doing OK for now, but October has been a terrible month for me. I took something called Cholestin, a herbal is for high cholesterol. I did not think it would harm me, but boy did it ever. I took a dose, and the next morning I started having lots of seizures. I had about eighty seizures in two days and the left half my face got numb and I also lost the ability to talk. That was a reaction to the drug, but it also caused a serve gall bladder attack. I spent four days in the ICU and one day in a regular room at the hospital, then one day for laser surgery at another hospital. They moved my gall bladder and found more than forty gall stones. Now I know that the abdominal pain I had over the past year was my gall bladder! I had no idea. But now I am doing OK and other than two to three seizures a week, I am feeling better.

I enjoyed the article you sent and thank you for it! It was really very interesting. I tried those research medications and many others, too. Sometimes I felt like a drunk and other times the medication would make me wonder if I were crazy because I would have weird thoughts and do strange things. Still, most of the time when I took Tegretol I was like in a shell, having panic attacks just about every time I left the house. Yet a lot has changed since they put me on Klonopin (Clonazepam) and Neurontin.

You are right about how hard is it for others to grasp what epilepsy can do to a person. We cannot give up or let it get the best of us! My philosophy is just like yours. The support group I started has helped me just as much as it has helped others. Thank you for saying such kind things about me. Expressing my true emotions is easy for me, especially in writing. You seem to be a very warm, thoughtful person yourself.

I believe this epileptic struggles, but her philosophy to cope with epilepsy helps her. Her ability to express her emotions verbally with others is helping her become stronger. Expressing yourself verbally is important because you can not hold your feelings of having epilepsy inside. You need to share your feelings with others so you can heal yourself and get on with your life.

Dear Stacey,

How are you? Last evening I had a seizure in the bathroom. I fell against the bathroom tub. We do not use the tub in our house. The tub is covered with a board and a rug is on top of it, so I do not fall really hard against the bathroom tub.

When I was younger, the doctor had put me on Dilantin. I would act crazy. Once when I was a child I put a wasp down my brother's back. He got stung. I got punished and now have a fear of getting stung myself. I did things like kick mud on my grandmother's leg. I wet my pants. I was nine years old at the time in school. The teachers would punish me and I would have to stay in for recess. I hardly ever got to go out for recess. I got to the point where I never wanted to go to school.

Now I do not have to take Dilantin that gave me those side effects. That medication would make me sleep all day. I also gained a lot of weight from the medicine, and I had a weight problem when I first became epileptic. Now, I go on six mile long walks every day. When I took Dilantin I felt dizzy. When I would go upstairs, I would have to hold on to the walls to keep my balance. I hit my mom; I quit hitting her once I got off Dilantin. I took Dilantin for thirty years. My parents and my brother thought that the way Dilantin made me act was normal. When they changed my medication, my family found out that they were wrong! I noticed my personality change for the better. I am forty-one years old and got epilepsy at the age of seven years old.

I believe medicine can do a lot to you're your body both mentally and physically. If for any reason you feel that the medication you take for seizures is making you feel or act funny, you should approach your neurologist immediately. If you do not like what your doctor has to say than you should get a second opinion. Never give up hope.

Dear Stacey,

Hi!, How are you doing? I am thirty-one years old. I have had epilepsy since I was five years old and am on Dilantin and Neurontin. My seizures seem controlled now.

I have a story to tell. It started January 1, 1984. I will never forget it. I was in a snowmobile accident. My friend drove up to the water plant at the dam, then told me to drive back. Like a fool I did. I was all right driving straight, but the road turned, and I went into a seizure and twisted. I rammed into a tree and. flew 10 feet. My friend moved me. I got a compound fraction of my spine, and lucky, I'm not in a wheelchair. A tree branch almost poked my left eye out. It gave me a scar. I knocked my four front teeth out and had to get a plate. God was watching over me. I do not drive anymore. I use a bus to get where I have to go. My husband helps too. He brings me where I want to go. I do not want to hurt myself or anyone else. I got off easy.

I used to live with my parents and they took good care of me. When I got married, I thought things were going to be different. I thought I could get my license and could drive and thought I could focus on my career. Things did not turn out that way.

Someday I hope things can be different. For now I need people like you in my life. Then someday I can turn my life around. I have the Epilepsy Foundation in my life. My therapist is teaching me many things. Then my husband is a sweetheart. He is a big part of my life. I am glad that I met him and that we fell in love with each other.

I hope that my story can help other people. Like you said, "there are different cases out there." Take care and God bless.

I think this letter shows you the importance of love and support. You cannot cope with epilepsy by yourself. You need the help of others. Never feel embarrassed or ashamed to reach out. Even the people without epilepsy need the help of others to survive.

Dear Stacey,

I am a 46-year-old single bachelor. I have epileptic seizures for the past forty years so far. My seizures started in New York City, when I was playing ball on the street with the other boys that time. I was the only six years old on June 1959. When I tripped and hit my head against a large rock. When I came home, I did not really feel that well. I began to get seizures one after another.

My parents had to call our family doctor and he came over to our home and he looked at me. He said, "Michael is having epileptic seizures." So he called an ambulance to have me admitted to Columbia Presbyterian Medical Center. I had to stay in the hospital for two weeks and they did many tests on me. The doctors tried all kinds of medicines on me, but none of them controlled my seizures at all. The only medication I am taking is Dilantin 150 mg. , Phenobarbital 100 mg. , and Valruim 50mg.. I have been taking these medications for the past twenty-nine years, since 1957 to June of 1986. A year or two later, I went to my new neurologist in Kingston, New York. He did many experiments on me. Then the FDA in Washington, D.C. approved more new drugs and my physician had prescribed me Depakene (Valproic Acid) 250 mg., and Tegretol (Carbamazepine) 200 mg. four times a day. These medications help get my seizures under control and I feel just great. I have been taking these medications for eleven years so far.

I believe this man did not give up hope. He kept trying to find that wonder drug that would help him become seizure-free. Through his strength and determination, he was able to find the right drug for himself.

Dear Stacey:

How do I feel about having epilepsy? When I first started through all the MRI's and the EEG's, it was scarey. Still, to know what you're really dealing with is less scarey. At least, I know it was not a brain tumor. I think anyone with epilepsy just needs to remember we need to practice discipline in our lives. If your life has no discipline you are in much trouble if you have to deal with epilepsy from day to day. I never thought of myself as a discipline person til I had to deal with having epilepsy and I learned how disciplined I was or maybe how disciplined I have to be! My sketching is really therapy for me. I can sit and do it for hours. I am no great artist, but it relaxes me. I go back to the doctor the end of October and we will see where I go from here. I feel sure my doctor will want to change the dosage of my medication.

Take care and again it was good hearing from you.

I think everyone needs some type of discipline in their lives. Discipline helps us put our life into perspective. You need a clear mind to focus on your mind, body and spirit. You need to understand yourself so you are able to develop inner peace with yourself and have clear direction on where you're going in life.

Dear Stacey,

Hi! How are you doing? I am OK. I was five when I came down with epilepsy, too. My seizures are under control with Dilantin and Neurontin; thank God. I have Grand-mal seizures where I shake all over. I do not feel so good before and after a seizure. I know when a seizure is going to come.

It sounds like you do not let your epilepsy run you. It sounds like you're a happy person. My friend went for surgery. She has been seizure-free for a long time. I asked my doctor about surgery and he said that I did not need it. He said, that my seizures are OK. I was terrified about it too. You do the best you can; that's all you can do.

Well, I am going to go. Take care and God Bless.

What I liked about this letter is that this epileptic said, "you do the best you can; that's all you can do". You don't have to prove to anyone who you are and what you're capable of doing. What you need to do is make sure is that you're happy with yourself that's all that matters.

Dear Stacey

I hope you and Michael have a happy Valentine's Day and that life is treating you well. I would give anything to have 2-3 seizures a month, consider yourself lucky in a way. I have been having so many I lose count. Nevertheless, I am happy to hear that you are doing better.

It is good that you are willing to stay on the drug study; more research does need to be done. I hope God will be with you and your baby, so that everything will be okay. I took Tegretol for about ten years and it did not control my seizures-but the doctor would not change it. It caused me to have panic attacks and I was afraid to be around people. Nevertheless, I came off it last year and my family said, that my personality has really come out now! Mentally I feel so much better. I am on Neurontin and Klonopin and still have poor seizure control.

Also, the past few days I have had a virus and ran a fever- that makes my seizures worse. Since I cannot take cold/flu medicines, I have been taking some herbs that are helping some. I quit going to V.A. for a neurologist, because of mistreatment, in the way of prescribing med. that conflict with each other and sent me into seizure clusters. So now I go to a neurologist who specializes in epilepsy, one the Epilepsy Foundation recommended. She is really good and will have me monitored in the hospital for a few months.

Keep me informed on how your pregnancy goes. I know a married couple who *both* have epilepsy and take lots of medicines, yet have three healthy children, which should be encouraging to you. Keep in touch. In love & friendship

I believe this epileptic received medical advice through the Epilepsy Foundation. The foundation offers many things to people who have epilepsy. Also, this letter tells us to have strength, stay strong and don't give up hope. Our prayers will be answered.

Dear Stacey,

I was at my daughter's dentist the other day. She is back from her maternity leave and was showing me pictures of her baby. She told me to tell you that if a woman of thirty-nine with epilepsy can make it, you will too. It is her first baby, she said, she was really surprised that she did not even have a slight seizure while in labor.

Maybe now that you know you can stay on the Oxcarbazepine, your stress will be less. I just think it is great that your EEG shows your seizures are better. I went to the doctor's last week. Well by the time she walks in and sits down, I have a major seizure, get rigid and cannot talk. I have not had one like this in ages. She immediately orders an EEG. She was on her way to lecture and I got the "pleasure" of talking to a neurosurgeon. He told us about strip surgery on the brain or VNS. My dad was in the room with me and when he left, we both shook our heads. I am not ready for this and did not feel comfortable with it. I went home, prayed about it, and decided it's not what I want right now. When I get to the point where I cannot live with my seizures, then I may reconsider. Yes, my seizures have worsened. My doctor is taking me off some of my medications because I feel so drugged. I am getting ready to go to my medical doctor for a hormone checkup. I wake up in the night and I do not know whether it's "hot flashes" or the seizures waking me up. I sleep very little and that is not good for me. Naturally, with little sleep the next day I have seizures all days. Something's got to give!

I have a funny story for you. You know I sell Avon. Well, we have monthly meetings and last month a little old lady sat next to me during the meeting. She's close to seventy yrs. old and has been selling Avon for many years. We got to talking and somehow she mentioned that she took thirty pills a week. I told her I took 133. Of course, I explained that I have epilepsy. She said, that I did not look like that kind of person who had epilepsy and she was sorry for me. Well, I could not be mad at her because she was so uneducated about epilepsy and it gave us a little chance to chat and I told her a little more about it. I still think she felt sorry for me. I guess that really sweet, but it just goes to prove again how people do not know anything about epilepsy.

I love my doctor. Nevertheless, she does not have epilepsy and let's face it, she does not really know how I feel inside. Nor does she feel the same emotions associated with having epilepsy. I am sure they try to understand, but like I said before, she does not walk around with epilepsy, not knowing when she will be seized and have no control over it.

When you say something in a letter and it hits home, I stop and say I am okay she feels that way too. It is so easy to start to wonder if what you feel is almost not real, especially for me as an adult who developed epilepsy. Well, take care of yourself and the baby too. Your friend,.

I believe it is important for us to educate individuals who are unaware about epilepsy. Many individuals have many misconceptions about epilepsy. If we do not take the time out to teach the public about epilepsy then who will? This epileptic was able to have a baby. Epilepsy doesn't stop you from doing the things you really too in life, you just have to take good care of yourself.

Dear Stacey,

I have had a couple of bad seizures, one that really scared my husband. I remembered it started as an aura, but then on into a seizure. So my neurologist has put me on Tegretol XR (a time release version of the old Tegretol), which I have to take twelve hours apart. I think I am too worried about too many things, and this does not help.

I have psychomotor epilepsy. My neurologist of many years just looks at me over steeple fingers. Shaking his head, he tells me, "If the stress you are under because of your mother's affairs continues, you will continue to have health problems!"

My mother guarded the fact that I had epilepsy like some terrible secret! She never thought I should tell my friends I had seizures! My neurologist in

San Antonio, TX sent me off to college at Texas Tech in 59'. He gave me the instructions, "You must tell your roommate you have a seizure problem, and not to be alarmed, and what to do to help you. You must also tell aside your professors and caution to them not to be alarmed! I have always done this. It horrified her when I was on the Epilepsy Society Speakers Bureau. "Oh what will my friends think if they find out?" She cried to me.

I feel we all helped in the last thirty years to get epilepsy far out and beyond the old beliefs that people suffering from epilepsy were possessed by the devil or had some kind of evil spell cast over them! Lord, only knows it was hard going through school because kids did not understand what was wrong. My seizures were far more frequent and worse before I had brain surgery in 57'. The doctor says they missed a small section and that's what now causes my seizures. He says I need another surgery! Aloha,

I think this epileptic is a strong individual. She accepted the fact that she was epileptic and knew that she needed to use her experience with epilepsy to help others. She also had the strength to go through brain surgery. It's scary when you know someone is going to cut into your head and do a surgical procedure on your brain. Many thoughts cross your mind. What if something goes wrong? How will I feel afterwards? Will I be the same person that I was before the surgery? And most of all, she was able to handle her mother being in denial. It's very hard to go through life knowing that your mother doesn't fully accept you for who you are, yet that did not stop her. I am very proud this epileptic.

Dear Stacey:

How are you? I have had a cold the last week to ten days. I usually have more seizures during a cold. I had a reaction to a DPT shot when I was seven months old. I had a fever of a 100, with convulsions. I became epileptic when I was seven years old. The doctor traced the epilepsy back to the reaction (fever) from the DPT shot.

I took Dilantin for thirty years. It had the same effect as if I were to drink four beers. I use to hit my mom and I sat around half asleep lost in fantasy. I felt like a different person after they changed my medication. None of my family (including me) knew my actions were related to Dilantin. We all thought that was just the way I was. We found out different when they changed my medication.

I no longer have to wait until 2:00am for the hangover feeling (I felt like a drunk at the end of the day). I had to have both arms on the walls to keep my balance on our stairs. Come night I was never tired. I no longer have to live that way. I can put on my coat, my shoes and go for walks.

When I was in high school, kids that did not understand epilepsy made fun of kids that had epilepsy, even kids I knew since I was eight years. old. So when I go on my long walks I try not to worry about what will happen if I have a seizure on my walk. Most of the time nothing will happen.

I am the only member of my family that does not drive (because of epilepsy). Sometimes I wish I could drive, but on other days like today I put my coat, hat, and shoes and I went for a long walk.

I strongly believe that if you feel your body is not functioning right or you're personality seems to had change then you should go see your neurologist for some advice. Many epileptics have to go through many different anti-consultant drugs before they find the right medication. Any medication can alter the way you feel, think or act. Never be afraid to approach your doctor. Your doctor can not read your mind. You have to tell him how you feel. And there is nothing wrong with disagreeing with your doctor. You have a mind of your own.

Dear Stacey,

I have an average of four or five auras a month. I usually have auras due to stress. I have no children, but work with preschoolers since the 1970's. Down below I have listed things that have helped me with my epilepsy.

1. Seizures are not new. Mark 9: 17-29 tells of a boy who had seizures.

2. Famous people had seizures.

3. Working with preschool, who accept me for who I am.

4. I once had fear of who would see me have a seizure. Now I tell myself: stay calm and trust in the Lord.

5. I accepted Christ as my savior in 1959. I trust in the Lord and I have felt safe and secure since. I know there will not be any epileptics in heaven.

I believe you should hold these encouraging five statements in the back of your mind and think of them when you're feeling down.

This is a letter someone sent me telling me how they live with epilepsy.
Epilepsy in simplistic terms:
Don't get behind a wheel of a car. You could kill someone and yourself. If you drive, you put everyone that is on the highway in danger.

Don't take a bath or shower when all by yourself. You could die in a teaspoon of water. And drown before anyone would find you.

My experiences about having the disorder:

When I was in school, I told my friends that I had epilepsy. They said, I would never finish school, get married or have kids. I have done all three. I finished all in 1990 and had a perfectly healthy boy in 1992. I just got remarried this past November to a wonderful, good-looking man that loves me with all his heart. He can handle my epilepsy. I also have a wonderful stepson. I got remarried November 24, 1997. I proved I could do what they are capable of doing and sometimes better.

Having epilepsy: realizing you are not alone:

I had epilepsy since I was nine years old. When the doctors told me I had epilepsy I believed I was the only one that had the disorder. I started reading about epilepsy. I found out there was millions of people that had epilepsy. If you talk about your epilepsy, you will find out that you are not alone. You will discover that you can write and talk to people who have epilepsy that would love to help you and tell you about their experiences with the disorder.

Accept the disorder and learn to live with it:

At first, accepting that you have epilepsy seems hard, but I have learned to live with it in a positive manner. I put my faith in God and live day by day. I take time out of my busy day to thank God that I am healthy as I am, and for the things I do have: a wonderful husband and too little boys I love with all my heart. The three of them can handle my epilepsy. You will know who really loves you when they find out about your disorder. My friends and family helped me to think positively and not to give up.

These five things helped me to learn to live with my disorder in a positive manner:

1. Put your faith in God
2. Know you are not the only one with the disorder.
3. Set your goals high.
4. Be happy who you are.
5. Think positively.

I believe this letter talks about what I have been saying in this book all along. This epileptic has the right idea on how to cope with epilepsy and because she knows how to live with epilepsy, she was able to accomplish the goals she set for herself.

Dear Stacey,

I have been really busy taking care of my husband (he is finally back to work on light duty), helping my daughter get ready for college, tending to my Avon business and trying to find a little time for myself. (Training new reps for Avon that is a real trip in itself!)

I am doing much better now that I took it upon myself to modify my own medication. That is something I would normally never do, but it was that or go crazy! My doctor had increased the dosage of one of my medications. I felt like I was on a terrible drug high, or at least what I think one would feel like! My doctor was in Montreal for a week and I was talking with her head nurse and she was talking to the doctor each day about my situation. She was gradually reducing the dosage. Yet, it was not enough to help. The day came when the office was closed. The doctor was still in Montreal and I had the whole day to get through. That was it! Now my seizures are no better but, I had to live with that for a long time.

I am so excited about your book! It gives me a sense of pride to think that I might have made a small contribution to it. You know I may get down a little, but I pull myself back to reality and, like you, I know that I am not going to let epilepsy control me. I am bigger than that. Yes, I may have to change a few things in my life to live a little better with it. Still, I know that I can have a better quality of life by doing so.

I went to a seminar with a motivational speaker from Avon today. I am selling more and it has been a real hurdle for me to get over not driving, but I enjoy selling Avon and I decided I would do my very best. My business has really grown in the last four years. My manager passed around an article that was in the Woman's Day magazine at one meeting we have each month. So many women after the meeting were in awe that I would even sell Avon without driving. At that point, I would like to have made a little motivational speech of my own to tell them that you can do anything you want to do, when you put your mind to it. This is one for your book. Not to long ago, I was at my hair dressers and one of my customers who apparently did not know that I had epilepsy was there. She overheard another lady in the Salon ask how my seizures were and right aloud where everyone could hear she blurted out that she did not know that I had epilepsy. How in the world could I be on Avon Lady with epilepsy. Guess I was so astonished that I could not really even think of anything to say. Yet, that it was not a problem for me. I had a husband and daughter to help me get to my customers. I was really taken back!

I will continue to keep you in my prayers. Your most wonderful and happy years are ahead of you as you become a mom!

I like this epileptic's letter because even though she has a tough time with her epilepsy she does not let it get her down. She focuses on the positive things in her life and concentrates on making the people she loves the most happy. She also has her job which she enjoys and by molding her life the way she has; she has increased her strength, self-esteem and self worth.

Dear Stacey,

Ten years ago they diagnosed me with epilepsy. I was thirty, now I am forty-one. The medicines I am currently taking are Felbatol, Lamictall and Tegretol. Of course, I had tried so many medications before these. I used to take Phenobarbital, but it just did not seem to help.

I have the grand—mal and petite—mal seizures. My reactions are the same as yours, but my memory loss lasts a lot longer than yours.

I am so proud and thankful that you are writing this book. I have been through a lot since they had diagnosed me with epilepsy. My life before was an active life. I was never home. My friends would pick me up, since I do not drive and I would go out to eat or just hang out. Nevertheless, since I had a few seizures around them, they've stopped calling to go out. It seemed like I had a plague. I would embarrass them, but they would never say it to me. My co-workers were acting this way at first, but they helped me out by treating me like I was normal. Yet in 1995, my doctor finally demanded me to quit work. He said, that it was the stress that was causing my seizures. I really doubt that because everyone has stress in their lives.

It took me about one and a half years before I really got over the fact that I could not work any more. Of course the seizures returned every once in while. That's when I really started to write letters to the Epilepsy USA Newsletter. These people have really helped me out. I don't feel so alone. I have started planting a garden to help my self—esteem. It is working I just want everyone to know that I am not dead. I still can do things for my myself.

I am so proud of those that are still working. I just wish that I could work, but I have just placed my faith in the Lord and he will help me along the way.

My family had been very supportive of me. The only thing that I need to conquer is to going out to eat or shop. They are major things. Nevertheless, as I said before the Lord is helping me so, when I do go out I pray for his help.

Your friend,

I believe the Epilepsy Foundation can help any epileptic get their life back on track. When your seizures are occurring frequently it's hard to go about your daily activities. This could become depressing. Yet if you have support from other epileptics and individuals who can help you create a life suited to needs, then you can over come the obstacles put in front of you.

Stacey,

I am giving a lot of thought about doing something goofy. I would like to hike the entire distance of the Appalachian trail. I need to do something for me. I need to feel a sense of adventure flowing through my veins again. Since I had to stop working, I feel like I only exist. I feel like I am in a void and cannot break out. I do not know if I could get ready to go by next year, but it would be a fine way to celebrate my fiftieth birthday in the year 2000. When and if you have time, let me know your thoughts about it. If you know someone that made the hike, maybe you could connect me with them to get information on how to get ready. My doctor will probably flip out when I tell him my plans. I see him next month.

May God fill your life with peace and happiness.

I think its great that this epileptic is searching for something to fill his inner needs. We all have dreams, hopes and wishes. We need to always be aware of what of what are mind body and soul are trying to tell us. We always need to please ourselves because if we can't please ourselves than how can we make the people around us who we care about happy.

Stacey,

Hi, how is everything going? I am doing well over here. I am glad to hear everything is doing well with you and the baby. I had one seizure this month so far. I believe everything happens for a reason. When I got my divorce, I believed no one would marry me because of my seizures, but I asked God to send me a good man and he did. He is a great man.

It took me a long time to realize I was not the only one with seizures. Nevertheless, when I finally realized I was not the only one, I knew I could write to people who also knew how I felt. So far I have gotten much support from other people. These people really understand me, They are epileptic, too. I believe other people need to realize that people with seizures can do everything except drive and take showers by themselves. I have been lucky so far to have a wonderful man who loves me for myself, and who can handle my seizure disorder, and a wonderful son. I love all three with all my heart. That is all for now. I will be praying for you and your family. May God be with you all!

I think if you have determination and hope anything is possible. This epileptic through prayer and hope found herself a man that accepted her epilepsy and wanted to spend eternity with her. Through reaching out to other epileptics she was able to develop strength and a higher self-esteem. It is so important to understand that you are not the only one with epilepsy. Many individuals that have epilepsy go through the same thoughts, feelings and physical trauma as you do.

Dear Stacey,

It sounds like an exciting time for you and the baby. Sorry to hear you are still having seizures, but hopefully one day you will find the right medicine to stop them together. I still have seizures occasionally. Sometimes, it makes me feel depressed and sometimes it does not bother me at all.

I have not been feeling too good and cannot figure out what is wrong. I am anemic and this could make me feel bad. I am now on hormones and it can also make you feel depressed. It is always something!

How did you know you were having seizures? Are your seizures mostly frequent when you are sleeping? I agree with you about the support. We need to help one another-that the family does not fully understand. I lacked support groups, but could not find any close enough for me. Driving is my problem, as you know.

I respect you for not letting epilepsy get you down and you shouldn't. You are young, married and about to become a parent, and isn't that what life is all about!

I think when you have trouble reaching support groups because you are unable to drive, then you must reach out to others and ask for help. As friends or family members to take you to the support groups. If you are unable to get rides during the time of the meetings, then you have to look for other ways to help you and your epilepsy. Have the Epilepsy USA delivered to your home so you can find out about other events in your area or write to other epileptics. There are other epileptic addresses lists in the magazine. Call the Epilepsy Foundation and find out how you can become involved. There is always a solution.

Stacey,

Congratulations, how is your new little one doing? Last weekend I went on an epilepsy retreat. I met many people. We played volleyball, softball, made beads, went on a hay ride, practiced archery, climbed a wall. It was so interesting meeting people with all different types of epilepsy. Last week I was in the hospital for testing because I am really considering surgery. My medication is just not working. My seizures are found on the left temporal lobe. Now next week I had to have on MRI. done and a Grid test to decide where they are going to take the piece out that needs to be removed. We are not sure where we want to have the surgery done. That is what were investigating right now. I am so happy that my new boyfriend is staying by my side through all of this.

I think going on retreats is a good way to meet other people and develop self-confidence in yourself. Doing different physical activities is great for the mind, body and soul. It helps you realize that epilepsy does not stop you from living and enjoying the wonderful life that God has given us.

Dear Stacey,

Thank you very much for writing. I also have epilepsy. I do have the partial complex seizures.

I am twenty-three years old and started having seizures at the age of thirteen in 1986. I still have them to this day. I am now seeing a new Dr. and he is very wonderful. You mentioned that you could become pregnant.! They told me that I was never was going to be able to have children unless my seizures were 100% controlled. Well, I have not

had any luck. ! I have been with my fiancee for three years and no luck at all. We are planning to get married sometime this year or at the beginning of next year.

As for my medications I am taking Neurontin 400mg and Tegretol 200 mg. I just had Neurontin increased, so I am taking another. Together I am taking fifteen pills a day. Nevertheless, it is helping me a lot more. ! I have not had any seizures lately ever since they have moved my dose up! I have to go six months without having a seizure before I can get my driver's license. Well, we will see what happens.

I was on a much better medication before. ! I was taking Felbatol. I was almost to the point where I was close to getting my license then I read that it was not good for the body so then I went to my doctor and told her that I wanted to be off it. So they then put me back on Tegretol. Nevertheless, it is helping me for now.

Well I have to get going now. Take care and hope everything goes great with the baby.

I believe this epileptic had the right idea when they decided to switch medications. Every medication has its drawbacks. What matters is that you have to feel comfortable taking the drug. This epileptic was not pleased with the drug because of what she heard, so she took the initiative and approached her doctor.

Dear Stacey,

I am glad you are still on Oxicarbazepine.. It sounds like a good drug for you and the baby. I am so proud of you and how you held up through your pregnancy. If this drug is the one for you, by all means try to stay on it. I appreciate knowing that some neurologists help you with your research program. Your prayers are already said, girl. I have prayed for you, believe me.

I have some good news for you. I was having some bad seizures. Then the doctor put me in a clinic for eight days. They took all my medicines away from me, keeping me up to 2:00 A.M. and waking me up at 7 A.M.. I had a bad seizure, splitting my head open between my eyes. Now I am on Depakote and seizure—free.

God Bless,

I believe in order to reach our goals and dreams we need to put a sincere effort into what we want in life. This epileptic had a tough time with her epilepsy, but she had the strength to go into the medical clinic and go through extensive testing to help her epilepsy. She was also, able to achieve one of her main goals in life. She achieved her goal by being hopeful, using her religion to help strengthen her and having the ambition to succeed.

Chapter 2

EPILEPTIC POETRY

HAPPINESS CAKE

1 CUP OF GOOD THOUGHTS
2 CUPS OF SACRIFICE
1 CUP OF KIND DEEDS
1 CUP OF CONSIDERATION
2 CUPS OF YOUR THOUGHTS

Combine the ingredients and mix thoroughly. Flavor with love and kindly service. Fold in prayers, faith and enthusiasm. Spread all into your daily life. Blend with human kindness.
Serve with a constant smile and it will satisfy the hunger of many people less fortunate than ourselves.

Thank the lord,
For all of his mercy,
And love,
Amen

LOST IN THE FOG

They asked me to explain in a speech to the doctors
What my seizures was like;
And I knew I had to tell them,
It was far worse than falling off a bike.
Then suddenly I remembered
The balls of ground fog rolling down some distant hill,
That closed in over you like a blanket
And somehow seemed to dampen even one's own will.
And so I liken my seizure,
To this fog which does descend;
I know not the beginnings or the end
Of those lost moments in time.
For during this descending fog,
I might not even remember
What the time, the day, or week;
Or whether this month is May or December,
It does envelop me so.
But then the fog will clear,

And yet the time frame is forever lost.
Left like a soul wandering in the rolling fog,
Whose sense of direction has been tossed
Into the stillness of the brain's eerie, ghostly
And somehow it did seem to satisfy
Those physicians searching curiosity,
The need to have a patient to tell them,
This is what it is really like
When I have a psychomotor seizure
And I lose those moments in the fog,
Never to be regained in life!

BOTTLES IN A ROW

Pills, pills, pills
All those pills on the shelf;
Bottles filled with pills and more pills
I mutter to myself,
All my life, I've taken pills!
Pills, pills, pills
Since my childhood, take them I must.
For when my seizures came
The adults always fussed,
'Did you take your pills today?'
Always there were strange bottles,
Bottles filled with pills.
Through my life so many passed—
All designed to cure the ills
Of my seizures.
But none to cure the crushed spirit
Of a child who stood apart.
But, no matter how good the pills

Oh woe. The seizures still came.
And Then the doctors poked and probed,
With questions about who's to blame:
The child, the medicine, or the errant brain
From whence the seizures came?
Then pills, pills, and more pills,
New pills to stem the tide
Of those seizure storms.
The search for the perfect pill

To let me have a way to hide
My seizures from the world.
But time and doctors knives
Did somewhat bring to heel-
The beast which roared within me
To cause the pain that I did feel
From the seizures.
But there are still the bottles
That bear the daily number
Of doses to be taken
To keep beast of a lesser seizure remaining

In its restful slumber in my brain.

SECTION TWO

EPILEPSY & YOU HOW YOU CAN WIN THE BATTLE

Chapter 3

MOVING AHEAD

To accept epilepsy into life, you must look it at it positively and realize that there is no such thing as a perfect person. There is no need to feel a sense of embarrassment because you have epilepsy. Each day of our life that we try to master the daily troubles that come our way, and how to overcome the problems that have already occurred in our lives, should be considered a triumph. Ignoring your problems, not dealing with them, is the easy way out, to face them and deal with then are accomplishments. Accepting our problems and dealing with them helps us grow mentally, physically and spiritually. When I opened up, telling people about my seizure disorder, I was shocked to find out how many people had epilepsy or knew someone who had the disorder. I think one of our biggest drawbacks is that there is a lack of research on epilepsy and people do not speak about the disorder enough. Many individuals are uneducated about epilepsy and look at the people who have the disorder as weird or think of it as a disease. Obviously, both statements are untrue.

I believe God puts obstacles in our lives to strengthen us. When we are young, we have people in our lives that help to mold us. They help us develop the strength, wisdom and knowledge we need to survive in this world. Yet if we become dependent on these people, we cannot survive and live the productive life that God has given us on this earth to enjoy.

Everyone is put on this earth here for a reason. We need to pass on what we have learned along to others.

It is selfish and pure laziness to pity ourselves because we have epilepsy. You must learn how to cope with your problems so you can help who suffer from the same difficulty. You are not alone, if you feel you are unable to straighten out your life the way you want it to be.

To live with and accept epilepsy, you need to open your heart and listen to what it is telling you inside. Your heart will never lie to you because it only tells the truth. You must have the courage to ask your heart why you refuse to accept the fact that you are epileptic. Usually when we chose to hide things about ourselves, it is because we are embarrassed about whatever we are trying to hide. Epilepsy is not something you should be ashamed of having. People with diseases, and disorders are constantly coming out into the open. They are learning to talk about the problems in their lives and are educating society about them. This is the way they heal the scars inside them.

Society is becoming less fearful about many of the diseases and disorders that unfortunate individuals have to live with. There are more and more support groups and research studies. Nothing is going to get better for epileptics until we learn to help each other.

There are self-help groups for everything because people realize that to change and strengthen themselves they must accept what they have and learn how to live with it in a productive manner. You need to look at life in a positive way. You need to say to yourself, "OK, I'm not happy with the person, I have become. I need to change and this is what I am going to do about it." Stop being lazy. This is the first step to healing and strengthening our souls and self-esteem. Be proud in who you are. Be thankful each morning that you can wake up and feel the warmth of the sun and the beauty that surrounds us all.

Chapter 4

Your Inner Self

Each individual has their own beliefs. I believe that each individual's life is predestine and what I mean by that is that God plans our lives before we are born. I feel that everything is done for a reason. You need to love everything about yourself and realize that God does everything for a reason. We may not understand now, but eventually our questions will be answered. This does not necessarily mean that the answers will be laid out on the table for you, but eventually you will put together the pieces to the puzzle. Yet as time passes we can usually see things more clearly and comprehend why everything turned out the way it did. I feel that God walks with us during these troublesome times, and he gives us tools we need to get through these times. As these problems are occurring, we are learning also, so we can help others struggling. It is our decision to choose, if we are going to use the tool's Gods given us. Rejecting the options God has given us would be foolish because it will help better our lives and strengthen our inner souls.

Each individual is made up of three parts, the mind, body and spirit. We can do anything we put our minds too. The mind is a powerful and vital part of our body. Many underestimate its capability.

After talking to many epileptics, including myself I have come to the conclusion that our biggest downfall is accepting the fact that we have epilepsy. Most epileptics I have spoken to or received letters from expressed the embarrassment that they have experienced living with epilepsy. Some told me that their parents forced them to keep quiet about their disorder because they were different from other kids. Some people wrote to me and told me others tormented them in school. Many individuals had numerous seizures each day. They felt living a normal life was almost impossible. It was understandable why some of these people developed anger toward having epilepsy and became reluctant to accepting the fact that they were epileptic.

When I was young, I always felt like I had to prove that I was no different from anyone else. For example, when my doctor told me not to dive off any diving boards, I made sure I found myself the highest diving board to jump off. I wanted to prove that I was no different that anyone else. I never told anyone that I was epileptic because I was embarrassed of my condition. I realize now that I was foolish to hide the fact that I had epilepsy and that I should be proud of myself. Epilepsy is a part of me and if I am going to be proud of myself than I need to be proud of the fact that I have epilepsy.

You can learn to love yourself and accept your condition. Change comes from within the heart, if one wants to change then there is nothing from stopping you. The ability to change only comes if you want to change. If you do not change, that inner eagerness, the desire to want to change, the strength you need that comes from you mind, body and soul will not suffice. You will not heal and become the person you want to be. Make sure this is what you really want. For whatever reason, if you are unsure if you want to change than search yourself and find out what is stopping you from becoming a better person. Being afraid to change is normal. Change takes time and courage, to change we need to look at ourselves honestly. I am here to tell you that you can become the person you always wanted to be and feel proud of yourself.

Accepting that you are epileptic is the most important and most critical step in learning to live with your disorder. To live with a happy state of mind, you need to have high self-esteem. You need to feel that you are no different from anyone else and that you can be the person you set in your mind to be. You need to reconstruct your life. You need to put yourself in a lifestyle that will make you happy and bring you as little stress as possible.

Stress is the worst thing for an epileptic. Stress brings on seizures. Therefore, you most try to avoid stressful situations and try to live your life with as little stress possible. During the day if you feel you are becoming stressed, you should try massage therapy. This is when you relax the muscles, ease muscle spasms and pain, increase blood flow in the skin and muscles, relieve mental and emotional stress, and induce relaxation. You could also try listening to music to relieve stress or talk to someone about what is bothering you. Having a pet aids in reducing stress. If you tend to stress easily, you may want to give some thought to having an animal friend to help reduce your stress.

Learning to love everything about yourself is one major step in learning to accept that you have epilepsy. If we are unhappy with ourselves, then we need to change what makes you unhappy by going through the process of change.

The process of change involves several things. First let us ask ourselves, what does loving ourselves for who we are really mean? What does it involve? Is this something that is easy to accomplish or does it take time and effort? Learning to love ourselves is not easy and it does not happen overnight. Loving yourself takes time and this is something you must work at each day. You need to be able to get up each morning, and look in the mirror and like the person that you see. If you are unhappy with that person than you have to do something about it.

I have worked hard trying to change the things that I did not like about myself. It has taken me years of hard work to get to this point. I realize that I am no different from anyone else. I do not feel embarrassed of having epilepsy and have become the person I set forth to be. Nevertheless, the key to all this is living life with a healthy and productive perspective in, not a rebellious one. You must set reasonable goals and objectives in your life.

The first thing, I did to help me on my road to success was to say to myself aloud, "I am Stacey Chillemi and yes, I have a seizure disorder." You need to hear yourself say that there is nothing is wrong with having a seizure disorder, absorb it into your unconscious and conscious mind. Once you learn to strengthen your inner self and develop strong self esteem, you will begin to feel you can accomplish whatever you set your mind on. You must understand and truly believe that no one can change you; only you can change yourself.

I needed learned to love myself by accepting all my faults and putting the past behind me, but if you focus on your faults than you will only experience an unhappy life. You need to think positively and focus on your accomplishments. My life began to change for the better once I started to focus on my achievements and stopped dwelling on negative things. We all deserve to live life to its fullest.

To be able to live with a seizure disorder, you need to develop a great emotional strength strength so you can accept the negative things about yourself, yet want to change them.. To heal yourself you must focus on all your positive qualities. You must change the factors that lessen your self-worth. Doing so will help you live a happy and healthy life and make you feel that you can accomplish anything the world dishes out to you.

To begin the healing process we need to develop *strength, wisdom, confidence* and *knowledge*. If you can develop these qualities, you will achieve all your goals and dreams. But first you must focus on the goals and dreams you want to fulfill. I am going to teach you the true meanings of strength, wisdom, confidence and knowledge and how to obtain and use them. This process of change theory will help you live a happy life and you will not be ashamed that you are epileptic.

Understand that all these characteristics come from inside us. Have you ever heard the expression, "mind over matter?" It means learning to take control of yourself and the world around you by using the knowledge you have gained. To use your mind productively, you have to understand yourself. Those that do not let others take control of them because they know what is best for them. By developing and acting on these qualities, you can look at epilepsy in a positive way and not view it as the ruination of your life. It will be a part of your life that you need to take charge of and nurture. You cannot hide the fact that your epileptic, and should not. You must become proud of who you are and realize that you are not the only one with this disorder.

Now let us look at each individual characteristic separately.

Strength- the development of strength in the inner body begins in the mind. The inner body is our mind, soul and spirit. How we think and program our minds to work, helps us build mental, physical and spiritual strength. Our strength comes from how we feel about ourselves. The higher our self-esteem, the stronger we feel and in turn we can do more for ourselves.

I cannot even begin to stress the importance of having high self-esteem; it is the key to having mental, physical and spiritual strength. The first stage of developing strength is learning to love yourself and your life. You need to learn to be grateful of what God has given you. You need to let go of all those angry emotions inside. Holding anger inside yourself will not help you, it will only hurt you. The past is just that—over. There is no way of changing the fact that we have epilepsy. Yet, if you have the strength and motivation, you can make the present anything you want. Having epilepsy will **not** interfere with your life unless, you let it. So many people who have written to me, or people I have spoken to, felt angry because they have seizures. To free yourself that anger, you have to say to yourself, **"Yes, I am an epileptic. I accept the fact that I have epilepsy and that I am unable to change the past. Nevertheless, I can change my future because I love myself and refuse to hurt myself by drowning in my own self pity."** You cannot rely on others. You need to learn to rely on yourself.

You have to believe in yourself, develop a sense of pride in yourself. It doesn't matter what others think about you, what matters is how you think about yourself. God put us on this earth to love ourselves and others, not to hurt ourselves and take our anger out on others, who are usually on the people we care about the most.

Knowledge—is the second part of the process of change, it is another important factor in helping deal with epilepsy. Knowledge comes from experience from being open minded to suggestions others may give. We may not always agree with other people's suggestions, yet it is always wise to listen to what others have to say. Some individuals may try to be controlling and may get frustrated if we do not act on what they have to say. You should to set these people straight and tell them; I will listen to what you have to say; however, that does not necessarily mean I am going to agree with you. I have my own mind, too and I need to do what is best for me.

We learn from each other and we acquire knowledge from the world around us that we should pass along to others by helping them. We need to take our past experience and use it in our present life now, including the mistakes we have made in life. The mistakes we have made are where we get most of our knowledge that helps us become stronger individuals. What weakens us when we repeatedly make the same mistakes.

Don't pity yourself for the mistakes you made in life or imperfections. Studies have shown that people who have negative attitudes are more like to live chaotic lives. They are more likely to become mentally or physically ill with extremely debilitating or life threatening illnesses. Many people have a hard time focusing on the positive because they allow their negative sides to consume them.. I firmly believe that focusing on the negatives will causes seizures.

Say to yourself, OK, what have I learned from these mistakes or from my shortcomings. Taking what you have learned and using it to help others is the best therapy. When you help you feel a sense of accomplishment and self-worth. You are overlooking any negative characteristics because you're too busy focusing on helping others'.

Confidence- our confidence comes from our self-esteem. To have high self-esteem we need to feel good about ourselves, to get to this point in life you need to begin by starting to do things in life to make yourself happy by focusing on the future, creating direction in your life. Begin by planning short and long-term goals for yourself and confidence level will rise.

It worked fir me. When I started accomplishing some of my short term goals, I had more self respect. I developed a greater sense of pride and my inner strength and self-worth increased.

Wisdom- comes from your sixth sense. We all have five senses, our sight, hearing, smell, taste, touch, yet I believe wisdom to be our sixth sense. Wisdom is understanding the inner signals and the directions that your body send out to you, becoming aware of what your body is trying to tell you. Your sixth sense always leads you to the right answers. It is up to us to learn to understand our inner self (spirit) and to follow the signals it sends out to us.

Listening to what our inner self has to say is essential. For example, have you ever felt like you had a feeling something was the right thing to do. You need to learn to understand your mind, so you can understand your inner soul and all the wonderful things it is capable of doing. When we listen and act on the signals it gives us, we become stronger and to understand our body as a whole. Spiritually you can give your body what it needs.

We feed our body food to survive on a daily basis. Spiritually we need to feed our body with love, understanding and different forms of relaxation, such as meditation. I strongly suggest to everyone that they start with at least five minutes each day with some type of relaxation exercise. Either in the morning when you start your day, the afternoon if you are able too or at night before bed to release the tension that has built up throughout the day. Each week you should add five minutes till you get to hour each day.

When you do these things, you increase your level of strength, wisdom, knowledge and confidence. By having a high level of strength you feel as though you can conquer the world. This helps you decrease your stress level.

Once you accept epilepsy in your life, you can cope with the world around you and accept the fact that you can do everything you expected to do in life. But to accept that you have epilepsy you first have to love who you are and be proud of the person you have become. There are many things in life you are capable of doing, but you must develop the motivation and the will to get out there and **JUST DO THEM!**

Chapter 5

THE NEW YOU

Changing yourself mentally, physically and spiritually does not happen overnight. The process of change takes much time and energy, so do not get discouraged. While focusing on this program you will begin to see the changes in yourself as they start to occur. I felt exceptionally proud of myself when I saw myself begin to change for the better. My self-esteem improved and I no longer cared what others thought about me. For the first time I was concerned about what I thought, not what others thought. Believe me, once you begin working on this program you will begin seeing results and realize that this program is worth doing.

Remember, you cannot say you want to change, you have really to want it to do it. The motivation to want to change has to come from within your heart. Saying you want to change is easy, but you have really to want it to do it for it to happen. Otherwise, the change will never occur.

Below, are the **seven steps** to the beginning of the **transformation process**. The transformation process begins when you realize it is time to change and you finally develop the stamina to do what it takes to improve yourself. I created seven steps so that starting the program the right way will be easier for you. Your mind, body and soul all have to be on the same track, functioning as one or else the program will not work for you. The most important part of the program is the beginning. You have to have the correct perception of what you will be doing now and where you will be are headed for the future.

I used these seven steps myself to help me change my outlook on epilepsy. I was able love myself and not be ashamed that I was epileptic. I felt capable to live the life that I wanted to. I felt like a different, better person. I strongly believe that if you follow this program it will help to live *your* life as an epileptic proudly, creatively, and happily.

Below are the seven steps to lead you to a new beginning living with epilepsy.

STEP ONE:

STEP ONE **PATIENCE**—This is the first step to living a happy and healthy life with epilepsy is developing **patience**. You will need patience to work this program successfully. changing your outlook on epilepsy is going to take time, devotion and hard work. Succeeding with this program comes by being patient in wanting to see results.

This exercise will help you even if you are already a patient person because it will relax you and increase your motivational skills simultaneously.

1. Take a hot bubble bath for fifteen minutes. Also place an oatmeal bath in the water.

2. Lie in the bath tub and close your eyes, take four deep breaths slowly.

3. While your taking these deep breaths clear all thoughts from your mind. Focus on the feeling of the warm water touching your body and the breathing techniques that you are doing at that moment.

4. Think about something positive and pleasant. Envision something that makes you happy. Focus on something that makes you feel good about yourself.

5. Let go of any negative thoughts that you have stored in your mind. Just to think about one thing that makes you feel good about yourself.

6. Take four more deep breaths, relax for a minute and get out of the bath tub.

7. Get dressed, go to a quiet place and sit on the floor. Close your eyes and slowly bend forward, relaxing any tight muscles that are causing you tension. Bend to the left, stretching your arms as far as they will go, then stretch to the right, repeating the movement.

8. Take five more deep breaths and say aloud "I have the patience to change myself and become the person I want to become in life." Say, "I have epilepsy and there is nothing wrong with being an epileptic."

9. Repeat step seven and eight

10. Take five more deep breaths and listen to yourself when you're doing this exercise. Concentrate on yourself while doing this exercise. Do not let any distractions impose on your quiet time. Do not think about anything except this exercise and the techniques it involves.

Changing your outlook on epilepsy means. Not letting your epilepsy take control of you. As I was growing up, I always made believe that I did not have epilepsy. By doing this I was only hurting myself. Accepting epilepsy into my life has helped me tremendously. I have released much of the anger that I held inside myself, and have focused on other parts of my life, as a result I have become a stronger person, extremely proud of the person I have become. You need to do the same. It may take time to get to this point. That's why you need to have patience to come to believe you can do anything you put your mind too. Thinking positive thoughts about yourself will help you get a long **way in life.**

STEP TWO:

Step two teaches you how to recognize all the wonderful things about yourself. Judging other people is very easy. Looking at ourselves honestly, however, is difficult. Sometimes we do not focus on ourselves because we have become so preoccupied focusing on everyone else that we forget number one. This step helps recognize all the good things about yourself. You will begin to have a more positive outlook on life. First you need to ask, "What do I have to change about myself?, What parts of my life need to be readjusted? What are my strengths? What are my weaknesses?

Before you answer these questions get yourself a notebook. to document your answers to these questions and keep track of your progress. The journal helps you see your characteristics and change the ones you dislike. Look at the positive things about yourself and commend yourself for the accomplishments that you achieved and work on changing the negative characteristics that we all carry within us. Begin the journal by listing all the positive things about yourself on the first page. Make a list that looks like the following.

THE POSITIVE THINGS ABOUT ME
Your Strengths
1.
2.
3.
4.
5.
6.
7.
8.
9.
10.

Your positive points are the strengths that will take you through life. Start your journal with these positive characteristics. about yourself. Seeing your strengths itemized in your daily journal will give you encouragement. Each day as you open this journal, you will be looking at all the good things about yourself that will give you motivation to make this program achieve your highest potential. On the next page, create a list and write down your weaknesses. Make a list that looks as the following. Remember, be honest with yourself and make sure you focus not only on your strengths, but on your weaknesses. Reviewing our weaknesses can help us see more clearly what has to be changed in your lives.

THINGS ABOUT MYSELF THAT I NEED TO WORK ON *Weaknesses*
1.
2.
3.
4.
5.
6.
7.
8.
9.
10.

On the next page, list ten goals you want to do this week to change your outlook on epilepsy and how you feel about yourself. This will help you gain some insight into what you need to start doing for yourself. Start planning what you want the new you to be like. Each time you accomplish a goal, put a star next to it. Write down the date of when you achieved the goal. Create a list that looks like the following:

MAKING THE NEW ME
Goals for The Week   *Date*

1. Wrote a letter to five people with epilepsy.   *   9/15
2.
3.
4.
5.
6.
7.
8.
9.
10.

Then I want you to list ten long-term goals of what you want to have accomplished and where you want to be in a month's time. Focus on how your going to accept your epilepsy, be proud of the person you have become and how your going to change the characteristics about yourself that you do not like. **Make the list look like the list I have created below:**

CREATING THE NEW ME

Goals for The Month

1.
2.
3.
4.
5.
6.
7.

8.
9.
10.

Create a page in the beginning of the book called the **priority calendar.** Ask your self these questions.

Priority Calendar

What do you regret not having made more time for?
1.
2.
3.
4.
5.
6.
7.
8.
9.
10.

If you had more time, what would you do with it?
1.
2.
3.
4.
5.

6.
7.
8.
9.
10.

What are the top ten priorities in your life right now?
1.
2.
3.
4.
5.
6.
7.
8.
9.
10.

What are your family-related goals?
1.
2.
3.
4.
5.
6.
7.
8.
9.
10.

What are your business goals?

1.
2.
3.
4.
5.
6.
7.
8.
9.
10.

In the back of the journal, take a quarter of the notebook and title it your **Daily Diary**. Dedicate the diary to someone you care about and feel close too, someone who would be proud to see you accepting that you have epilepsy and living the life, you want to lead. Dedicating the journal to someone you care about gives you motivation to want to change for the better. Write about the goals you accomplished and explain how it made you feel to reach them. Write about these achievements are making you into a better person and how their helping you with your epilepsy. Describe what you had to do to achieve the goals.

Date

_____

_____

_____

Date

_____

_____

_____

STEP THREE:

Step three is about the importance of self-determination and how to develop it within yourself. Self-determination requires that you make an agreement with yourself and keep it. You must have faith in yourself that you're going to do anything that you put your mind to. Your motivation to accomplish this program will become easier as each day goes by. Saying you're going to improve is easy, but you cannot just say your going to improve; you have to get out and accomplish the goals that you have set for yourself. You can't accomplish too many goals in one day. Changing takes time and as step one says, "You need to have patience." Try to accomplish one goal a week at first. Maybe two goals, if you have the time. Then accomplish another goal each week until you get to ten goals. These goals do not have to be difficult. You can set several little goals maybe only one large one. Working on yourself can be tough if you have a busy schedule; nevertheless, don't let that stop you. You have to make time for yourself. Remember; you come first in life. You need to believe that you are the best. You cannot take care of the people who mean the most to you or do the things in life that you want to do, if your mental, physical and spiritual well-being is not intact and strong.

STEP FOUR:

Reward yourself every time you achieve a goal. Your achievements are important and you should not treat them lightly. For example, take in a movie or reward yourself with some quiet time to relax and focus just on yourself. To me there is nothing better than having sometime alone with yourself. Do something that makes you happy. Remember, you cannot make others happy until you are happy with yourself.

STEP FIVE:

In your journal, make a list called **Record of Successes** and itemize all the achievements that you've accomplished. Create a list of everything good you believe you have done for yourself. This will make you feel good about yourself. For example, include the following:

RECORD OF SUCCESSES THROUGHOUT MY LIFE

My Achievements
1.
2.
3.
4.
5.
6.
7.
8.
9.
10.

RECORD OF SUCCESSES DURING THIS PROGRAM

My Achievements

1.
2.
3.
4.
5.
6.
7.
8.
10.

STEP SIX:

Develop a special time in the day for quiet time. Studies have shown that individuals who have a daily quiet time are less likely to become ill, and heal faster from illness than those who do not. Take a few minutes during the day to write in your journal. Try to make it the same time each day. Perhaps when no one is home or just before you start the day in the morning. You could also wait till everyone goes to sleep so that no one will bother you. Give yourself at least fifteen minutes to a half hour. Relax, and while you are writing and relaxing ask yourself the question; "Where am I headed in life and where do I want to be a year from now?" Then write about it. Make sure you're focusing on the things you want to accomplish in life.

The only way you will succeed in this life is making sure that epilepsy does not control your life. You need to feel proud of the changes you're making with this program. Focus on what you have accomplished. Think about how you feel about having epilepsy while writing in this journal.

The goal is to let yourself open up and write intimately and honestly about how you feel. This method helps heal your wounds so you can get on with your life. You have to learn to understand why you have reacted the way you have about having epilepsy. Think of ways to strengthen yourself spiritually and emotionally. Make sure you do not limit yourself because you feel sorry for yourself because you have epilepsy. That is self pity and it is unhealthy. You will never get anywhere in life if you pity yourself. Free yourself from any walls you have built around yourself. This program will help you do that. Become the person you were meant to be.

STEP SEVEN:

Now repeat the seven step process each day. Once you complete the seven steps go back and review the things you have written in your journal. These steps are a new way of life. Keep doing these seven steps each day till you get to where you want to be and you have become completely satisfied with yourself. There is so much knowledge out there for us to learn. It is there for anyone who wants it. I always add more goals to my list. You should always work on bettering yourself. Everyone is special everyone has something unique about them. It is your job to find out what those unique qualities are in you and how to make them work for you.

Chapter 6

BEING HONEST WITH YOURSELF

The only way to succeed in this program or in life is to be honest with yourself. Have you been trying to hide the fact that you have epilepsy all your life? If so It's time to let go of your fears, your shame and accept who you are. If you have been carrying many angry feelings inside yourself because you are angry about having epilepsy than you must rid yourself of those angry feelings. Often when we carry angry feelings inside ourselves we take them out on those around us. We also hide our weaknesses and the things we do not like about ourselves from others, hide them and also from ourselves. As a result, all the negative characteristics and emotions that we do not fix now will eat away at us little by little, and the person who suffers the most is you. Be honest with yourself so you can heal your old wounds and begin a new way of eye with a clean slate.

Lying to yourself and to the people around you will get you nowhere in this life. You will get farther in life by being honest with yourself and others. There is no such thing as telling little white lies. One lie leads to another lie, and the lie grows bigger. Being honest with yourself is not something you do just in this program; you must be honest throughout your life.

You have to be proud of yourself. If there is something about yourself, you are not happy with than you need to change it. To do that, you must be honest with yourself.

Epilepsy is a part of your life. It won't disappear, so you need to learn how to live a fulfilling life. Understand that you are not alone and that there are many individuals with the same disorder who are eagerly looking for support. Epilepsy should not stop you from accomplishing what you want in life, unless you let it.

Our main goal is to repair all the emotional and psychological damage that we have inflicted upon ourselves over the years that have been harmful to our mind, body and soul. Say that, "I am not going to hurt myself like this anymore. I am too good a person for this." You are who you make yourself to be. To feel better you must free yourself from all the negativeness that you stored inside yourself and fill your soul with peace and serenity.

You cannot and should not blame anyone for being epileptic. Rid yourself of any resentments you maybe carrying, toward yourself. And thus. Make epilepsy a part of yourself. For many years, I have kept this saying in my mind maybe it will help you:

God grant me the serenity to accept the things I cannot change
The courage to change the things I can
And the wisdom to know the difference

Chapter 7

THE TRUE MEANING OF DREAMS

Dreams are the pathways to our inner souls; that come from our subconscious mind. While we are sleeping, our body tries to send us messages about the wants and needs our body longs for. A person's dreams can give a sense of direction in life. Although we do not remember most of our dreams when we wake up they still have an impact on the way we think and function. Sigmund Freud believed that dreams are expressions of unfulfilled wishes and desires. Dreaming plays an important role in our lives. Speaking for myself, dreaming always helped me escape from reality to a faraway make believe world where no one could hurt me.

Studies have shown that people who are repeatedly awakened at the beginning of dream periods for several nights become irritable and have difficulty concentrating. If your body's natural sleep cycle has been interrupted and has been deprived of dream sleep, your body will compensate by providing proportionately more dream sleep at the next dream sleep opportunity. Research shows that a healthy sleep is needed for a person's body to restore itself. Some scientists believe that adequate dream sleep is equally important because it enables the brain to recharge. Medical research has not proven this testimony. Usually, when a person is awake, their brain waves will show a regular rhythm. When a person first falls asleep, the brain waves become slower and less regular. They call this sleep state non-rapid eye movement (NREM) sleep.

NREM sleep consists of stages. There are four stages and each stage is a progressively deeper stage. The deeper the sleep, the more your body restores itself. Stage one sleep is the transition from wakefulness to sleep. Restoration begins in stage two, but is more significant in stages three and four, sometimes called delta sleep.

After an hour and a half of NREM sleep, the brain waves begin to show a more active pattern again, though the individual is in a deep sleep. This sleep state, called rapid eye movement (REM) sleep, is when dreaming occurs. A person typically experiences a brief arousal from sleep and returns to stage two sleep after dreaming. This sleep cycle has begun again. The length of time in each of these stages differs throughout the night, with most REM sleep occurring during the later sleep cycle.

Dreaming and fantasizing give you a feeling of serenity and inner peace. Fantasizing has a positive impact on you and your body. When you fantasize, you put yourself in a state of consciousness that lies between reality and the world of dreams. The imagination roams freely, although usually guided by mostly unconscious urges, concerns and memories. Fantasies help us find out what type of ambition we have and the people we want to become in life; it takes us into another world where we can do and become anything we want. It allows us to relax and joyfully think about the various scenarios that would make us happy.

While growing up, I always enjoyed sitting closing my eyes and fantasizing about something relaxing trying to analyze how my body was feeling the same time. It seemed when I understood my body and mind; I was able to make them function as one and then release all negative thoughts and feelings that were putting unnecessary stress on me. (Remember, the less stress you have the better for your epilepsy and seizure control.) My stress level decreased sharpen and so did the total amount of seizures I was taking monthly.

During this time of dreaming and fantasizing, you can focus on anything you want, including making goals for yourself on how your going to live your whole life having epilepsy. I have always dreamed about positive things. I knew I was going to survive having epilepsy because I refused to think negatively or feel sorry for myself. I looked at myself as a fighter and an achiever. I was not going to let anything get in my way.

Dreams can stay in your mind, no one has to know about them, and you can record them, in your daily diary, where you write down your significant dreams and fantasies. These dreams and fantasies can be used as motivators to help you work on accepting epilepsy in your life and learning how to live with it. Your dreams and fantasies can help you plan your life five or even ten years from now and you can use your dreams to strengthen your inner self. When life seems too stressful to handle; close your eyes and let your mind take you somewhere you can relax and fantasize.

Dreams are the pathways to your inner soul and it is your soul that knows what your mind and body needs. Reach out and get in contact with your soul because it is necessity that you take the time out to understand what your mind and body crave.

Keeping a journal has been a very successful tool for myself. I write everything down on paper from my short-term goals to my long-term goals, to my dreams and fantasies. This helps increase my inner strength by keeping me in touch with who I am and what I need to do with my life. I write down everything about the exams I take, about switching my medicines and anything else that's important to me. By writing everything down expressing how I feel I can understand myself better and the needs of my body mind and soul.

These are exercises you do in your journal will help you strengthen and understand yourself, and make you feel better about yourself as a person.

MY DREAMS

Date

WHAT THIS DREAM MEANT TO ME

HOW WILL I USE THIS DREAM TO MOTIVATE ME?

MY FANTASY

Date

WHAT THIS FANTASY MEANT TO ME

HOW WILL I USE THIS FANTASY TO MOTIVATE ME?

Keep a list of the dreams and fantasies you have that mean something special to you. Write down how they can motivate you in this program and how they relate to helping your epilepsy.

Do they relax you? Do they help you understand yourself better as a person? Do they give you hope for the future? While you write in the dream portion of your journal, answer the questions above. This is another way to strengthen yourself and understand your personal make up. These exercise will help strengthen your mind, body and soul in many ways.

Chapter 8

LOOKING AT EPILEPSY
IN A WHOLE NEW LIGHT

You have now helped yourself regain a new life by accepting that you have a seizure disorder and not letting it affect you. Major changes are occurring; spiritually you should feel like a new person, the person you have wanted to be for so long. By devoting time and effort to this program you have now taken the first step to feeling better about yourself. You should be beginning to feel that you can do whatever you put your mind too. You should be no longer ashamed of having a seizure disorder. Talking about epilepsy and telling others that you have the disorder should be easy for you now. You should be at the stage of where you are proud of who you are. You should have a clear outlook on how to live an enjoyable life with epilepsy as a part of it. You should no longer feel that epilepsy controls your life. You should feel enthusiastic about going after the goals you have set for yourself.

You have now become a stronger individual, with a more positive outlook on life. The negative characteristics (weaknesses) about yourself that you did not care for are slowly starting to disappear. This should make you feel proud and help boost your confidence and self-esteem.

You can succeed in this program, if you take the inner strength that you have developed it to focus on the positive things about yourself. Stop yourself if you begin feeling depressed because you have epilepsy. Dwelling on the fact that you have epilepsy will only end up ruining you, not helping you. Instead create a mental diagram in your mind on how you want the new you to look, act and feel. This will make you focus on all the good things about yourself. Your battle with epilepsy will be won when you conquer it with pride.

Another change I experienced was that I became determined to become seizure-free. I may not get that wish, but my drive to succeed in life grew stronger. I became more hopeful, more independent. I began to look at life from a more constructive point of view. I know I am going to succeed in life. Several years ago you would not have heard me say that.

As I started changing my lifestyle, I made sure that the people around me were a positive influence on my life. Sometimes the closest people around you are the ones that hurt you the most. I had to make sure that friends and family that surrounded me gave the respect and support that I needed. Are the people in your life loving or hurting you? If you want to help your epilepsy and control your seizures, you must be in a non-stressful environment.

It's vital to think of yourself as a high achiever and accomplish the goals in life that you always dreamed about fulfilling. Don't stop yourself from becoming the person you want to become in life. We all have are problems and we need to learn to work through them. Don't waste time and energy feeling sorry for yourself. Be tough and believe in yourself.

Chapter 9

THE IMPORTANCE OF
SELF-ESTEEM & SELF-CONFIDENCE

High self-esteem and your strong self-confidence will get you far in life. If you believe in yourself then you can succeed in anything you put your mind to. You may not succeed the first time you try, but you have to keep trying till you do succeed. You are too good a person to let yourself get to that point. God has blessed you by giving you a life to live, now you need to make the best of it. People give up hope when they attempt new methods and programs because they do not improve quickly. I have learned from my own experience and from others whom I corresponded with that. When you keep trying and you feel you're still not ahead of where you have started, you begin to lose hope for a seizure-free life. Quick success does not exist in our society. This is when you need to use your strength and tell yourself to stop, that you are not going to hurt yourself anymore. I battled with myself; sometimes I felt like I was winning the battle and at times I felt as though I would never make it over the hump, until one day I said, "no more," I was not going to feel like this anymore. From then on my life had a drastic turnaround. I became determined to become a new person, filled with hope, who was going accomplish anything I set my mind to do.

Achievements only come to those who strive hard to get them. You get nowhere in life if you do not push yourself. You need to create a lifestyle that is right for you and nobody else. Do not settle for anyone else's lifestyle or for a lifestyle that's beneath your standards.

To make this happen, you must learn to accept who you, be proud of the person you are. Only then will you feel your self-esteem rise up to the skies'.!

If you're still feeling that you don't have what it takes to complete this program then write whatever is still making you feel like you are not worthy of yourself in your journal. Even after completing the other exercises, if you still face obstacles that are holding you back, write them down in the journal immediately. Ask yourself what is making you feel like you cannot get to the point in life you want to reach. Organize your journal to look like this and write your feelings on the topics I just mentioned.

YOUR SELF-ESTEEM & SELF CONFIDENCE

1.
2.
3.
4.
5.
6.
7.
8.
9.
10.

Remember the past is over; you can only change the future. Having expressed what is bothering you, what your holding you back, begin to think how you can change the way you feel. Go through your journal and look at all the positive things about yourself. Concentrate on your strengths and write about why you do all the good things you do for yourself and for others in the back of your journal. These are the reasons you should love yourself and have high self-esteem and self-confidence in yourself. Give yourself credit for everything positive you have written about yourself. Remember, you're somebody special.

Ask yourself the question, what level of self-approval you have I reached living with epilepsy on a day to day basis? I have listed seven levels. Each of these levels will help you see the daily progress that you are make with this program.

LEVEL 1-   accept yourself as an epileptic and learning to love yourself for whom you are a person

LEVEL 2-   understand yourself mentally, physically and spiritually

LEVEL 3-   learn to control your mind, body and emotions

LEVEL 4-   strengthen your inner self and make it apparent to others

LEVEL 5-   begin changing what you do not like about yourself

LEVEL 6-   notice the change in our self-esteem and self-confidence

LEVEL 7-   have a tremendous amount of pride in yourself

When I went to the neurologist he would tell me what I could and could not do. I would become very frustrated. I would think to myself, "leave me alone," you know medically what I go through, but you don't actually go through a seizure like I do. When I would come home, my dad would make sure that I took care of myself. I was so sick of being looked after, I just wanted to be left alone. I know they were looking out for my best interest, but I had enough.

When I finally accepted myself as an epileptic I saw myself change one hundred percent. I became proud of myself. I saw myself no different from anyone else. I take my medicine. Some people take antidepressants other people take vitamins during the day. When I accepted that I had epilepsy I accepted everything about me and loved me for who I was. This was the best thing I ever did for myself. I felt as free as the birds that fly in our beautiful skies.

I was no longer hiding the fact that I was epileptic and was facing my disorder head on. A heavy accumulation of stress, depression and frustration left my body. There is nothing wrong with having epilepsy.

Accepting that you are epileptic is the most important and most critical step in learning to live with your disorder. To live with a happy state of mind, you need to have high self-esteem. You need to feel that you are no different from anyone else. You need to reconstruct your life and create a lifestyle that will make you happy and bring you as little stress as possible.

Stress is the worst thing for an epileptic; it brings on seizures. Therefore, you most try to avoid stressful situations and try to live your life with as little stress possible. During the day if you feel you are becoming stressed, you should try massage therapy. This relaxes the muscles, eases muscle spasms and pain, increases blood flow in the skin and muscles and relieves mental and emotional stress, and induces relaxation. Also try listening to music to relieve stress or talk to someone about what is bothering you. If you tend to stress easily, you may want to give some thought to having a pet to relax you. Everyone goes through life having to deal with something. There is a chance that one day we can be cured. May that day come soon!

SECTION THREE

HOW KEEPING YOURSELF IN GOOD HEALTH CAN HELP YOUR EPILEPSY

Chapter 10

KEEPING YOURSELF IN GOOD HEALTH EMOTIONALLY, PHYSICALLY AND SPIRITUALLY

PHYSICALLY KEEPING YOURSELF IN GOOD HEALTH:

To keep your seizures under control, you cannot just pop a pill in your mouth and think that is all there is to it. You need to keep yourself healthy by eating right, exercising and sleeping properly. These are important factors in helping to control your epilepsy. Certainly the medication we take to control our seizures plays an important role in our lives, yet if we do not take care of our bodies, we could cause ourselves to have seizures.

We need to try to take the best possible care of ourselves emotionally, spiritually and physically. The way we take care of ourselves affects us in many ways. When I started to take care of myself physically, I began to notice an increase in my energy level. Before then I was lacking energy, feeling fatigue and feeling sleepy. When I started to focus on my health and began to take better care of myself, I felt more emotionally stable and spiritually in touch with myself. I understood myself even better than when I began the program. I felt so proud of myself. Physically I looked like a new person and spiritually I felt like a new person. My self-esteem rose immensely. By feeling and looking healthy you begin to see yourself as a desirable individual about whom who you can feel proud. Once you start to feel proud of yourself, you will begin to feel like no task is too hard for you to achieve.

I began to realize the importance of keeping myself in good health and how my health was affecting my epilepsy when I went to see the neurologist one day. I was feeling fatigue and sluggish. My doctor told me that I was overweight for my height and built. I was twenty-two, five foot two and 146 pounds. The neurologist said, If I lost the weight I would feel better about myself both mentally and physically. By losing the weight I would help overcome my fatigue and help my epilepsy. My doctor had also mentioned that if I lost weight, most likely the doses of medicine I was taking to control my seizures would decrease. Personally, I was unhappy with my physical appearance. At this point, I realized that I could no longer let myself get any heavier.

The first thing I did to help myself get physically back into shape was change my eating

habits. If I were going to lose weight and get back into shape, I needed to change the way I consumed food. I love to eat, just like most people. I had an appetite for fatty foods, sweets, ham and eggs, cream cheese and other good foods that are not so good for the body. Pay attention to what your eating and eliminate any foods that are unhealthy and do not agree with your body. Everybody's metabolism is different, so you need to eat healthy foods that work best for you. For example, my body reacts well to carbohydrates whereas my husband's body retains much water if he ingests too many carbohydrates into his system.

I began eating mostly proteins and eliminated fatty foods as best I could. You need some fats in your meal plan, but make sure they're the right types of fats. Be careful with the fat-free foods they have on the market. They may have zero fat grams, but the amount of calories could be just as bad as a fatty food with many fat grams in it. To make the fat-free foods taste good they use a lot of sugar, which causes you to gain weight.

If you are at a weight that you're content with, then you should continue to eat healthy to maintain that weight and to keep in shape. Everything you put in your body effects your epilepsy. You should try to stabilize the amount of calories you consume each day after you decide the amount of calories you want to eat.

(In appendix 1, there is a list of calories and fat grams to help you.)

I stopped eating any cheeses unless they were fat-free. I stopped using any types of breads or other food products that had a high fat content. The bad thing about bread is that, breads make you feel full. When it goes into your body, it turns into sugar and increase your appetite. Soon you become hungry and want to eat again. Chinese food is high in carbohydrates, and has the same effect. The calories keep adding up and the salt in the food makes you extremely bloated. You should read the food labels when you shop in a grocery store. I ate many fat-free foods that were low in calories. I made sure that the product I was buying had little sugar and sodium in it. This was step number one to getting myself back on the right track. I tried to eat as few fat grams as possible in a day.

Drinking water is an important step to eating healthy. I made sure I drank as much water as my body could consume, which is important. You're trying to get your body back into shape and lose weight Water helps you flush all those unwanted impurities out of your system. The human body contains fifty to 70% water. Because water does not remain stored in the body, we must replace it continually. Water contains no fat grams or calories and is one of the healthiest fluids to drink. Adults must consume two to three liters of some form of liquid each day.

When I became hungry during the day, I made sure I ate healthy snacks such as bananas and yogurt. I cut out all the bad foods, such as the chips, ice cream, cakes, etc. I would have healthy meats such as chicken and turkey. Meats contain many valuable nutrients, among them is protein. But be careful also because meat also contains cholesterol.

I cut down on the mayonnaise, ketchup and all the foods that put on weight and hold water. It helped also when I ate slowly. By eating slowly I would enjoy the meal more and not eat as much.

I made sure I also ate breakfast in the morning. I noticed that when I did not eat breakfast, I would eat more during the day or at dinner time. You want to avoid eating big dinners because the food lyes on your stomach later in the evening and you do not burn as many calories. The food just lies there in your stomach. My daily diet consisted of a healthy breakfast, snack, lunch and dinner and a light snack. I felt fulfilled and I also lost thirty pounds!

Losing the weight helped me because I was able decrease the medication I was taking. After I began to lose weight my urge to eat decreased and I felt better about myself emotionally and physically. My body was feeling better and spiritually I felt my inner self began to feel at peace.

The Different Food Groups
Fat Oils and Sweets
Milk, Yogurt and the Cheese Group
Dry Beans, Eggs and Nut Group
Vegetables and Fruit Group Starches,
Grains, Pasta, Rice, Bread and Cereal

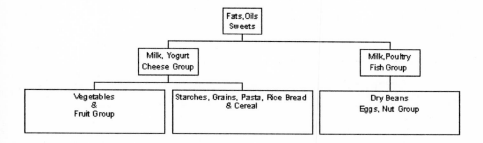

The bread-cereal group includes all breads and cereals that are whole-grain, enriched, or restored. All cereals are very high in starch, and they are good, generally inexpensive sources of energy. The fat content of cereal products generally is very low unless the germ is included. Whole-grain products contribute significant quantities of fiber and such trace vitamins and minerals as pantothenic acid, vitamin E, zinc, copper, manganese, and molybdenum.

Most vegetables are important sources of minerals, vitamins, and cellulose. Certain vegetables, such as potatoes, contribute appreciable quantities of starch. Large amounts of the minerals calcium and iron are in vegetables, particularly beans, peas, and broccoli. Vegetables also help meet the body's need for sodium, chloride, cobalt, copper, magnesium, manganese, phosphorus, and potassium. Carotenes (the precursor of vitamin A) and ascorbic acid (vitamin C) are abundant in many vegetables. Vegetables are useful as sources of roughage.

The nutritional value of fruits varies. Some fruits are composed largely of water, but contain valuable vitamins. The citrus fruits are a valuable source of vitamin C, and yellow-colored fruits, such as peaches, contain carotene. Dried fruits contain an ample amount of iron, and figs and oranges are an excellent source of calcium. Like vegetables, fruits have a high cellulose content.

The milk group includes milk and milk products, cheese, and ice cream. Milk is a complete protein food containing several protein complexes. It also contains important amounts of most nutrients, but it is very low in iron and ascorbic acid and low in niacin. Calcium and phosphorus levels in milk are very high. Vitamin A levels are high in whole milk, but this fat-soluble vitamin is removed in the production of skim milk. Riboflavin is present in significant quantities in milk unless the milk has been exposed to light.

The meat and meat substitutes group includes beef; veal; lamb; pork; organ meats such as liver, heart, and kidney; poultry and eggs; fish and shellfish; and dried peas, beans, and nuts. The meat group contains many valuable nutrients. One of its main nutrients is protein, but meat also contains cholesterol, which is believed to contribute to coronary artery disease. The minerals copper, iron, and phosphorus occur in meats in significant amounts, particularly iron and copper in liver. Different meats vary in their vitamin content. Liver usually contains a useful amount of vitamin A. Thiamine, riboflavin, and niacin, all B vitamins, occur in significant amounts in all meats.

Other Foods such as, butter, margarine, other fats, oils, sugars, or unenriched refined-grain products are included in the diet to round out meals and satisfy the appetite. Fats, oils, and sugars are added to other foods during preparation of the meal or at the table. These foods supply calories and can add to total nutrients in meals.

For many years the United States Department of Agriculture (USDA) issued dietary guidelines based on four basic food groups—meat and meat substitutes, fruits and vegetables, milk and dairy products, and grains, including bread and cereals—and a balanced diet would include at least one food from each group in each meal every day.

In 1980 the U.S. Department of Health and Human Services recommended that people eat a variety of foods daily, including fruits; vegetables; whole and enriched grain products; dairy products; meats, poultry, fish, and eggs; and dried peas and beans. While recognizing that certain people (for example, pregnant women, the elderly, and infants) have special nutritional needs, the report stressed that for most people the greater the variety of foods eaten, the less likely is a deficiency or excess of any single nutrient to develop.

The report emphasized that people should increase their consumption of complex carbohydrates—fruits, vegetables, and other unrefined foods— and naturally occurring sugars. It also recommended reducing the consumption of refined and processed sugars. It encouraged a reduction in fat consumption by decreasing the amount of fatty meats and replacing foods that have saturated fats with those having unsaturated fats. A reduction in the sodium intake by decreasing the amount of salt added to food was also recommended.

Research findings on nutrition, in the USDA and the Department of Health and Human Services changed the daily diet recommendations from the square of the four food groups to a food pyramid, with foods that should be eaten more often at the base, and those used less frequently at the top. The emphasis is on consuming less of the groups meat and meat substitutes, dairy products, and oils and fats, and more of the breads and cereals, and fruits and vegetables. When properly followed the food pyramid teaches the use of a wide variety of food items, moderation in total food intake, and proportionality among the food groups to ensure adequate nutrient intake.

Vitamins are carbon-containing substances that are required for normal metabolism but are not synthesized in the body. They are obtained, from such outside sources as food and water or are administered orally or intravenously. Exceptions to this definition include vitamin D, which is synthesized in the body to a limited extent, and vitamins B(12) and K, which are synthesized by bacterial flora in the intestinal tract. Minerals also must be obtained from outside sources. MineralsBsuch as calcium, iodine, and ironBare an essential part of all cells and body fluids and enter many functions.

Vitamins and minerals function as "cofactors" in the metabolism of products in the body. Most aspects of bodily metabolism proceed with the aid of specific enzymes, but if additional catalysts were not present—for example, the cofactor vitamins and minerals—the reactions would proceed so slowly that they would be ineffective.

Vitamin A has many important functions in the body that relate to membrane integrity, especially of epithelial cells and mucous membranes. It is also essential for bone growth, reproduction, and embryonic development.

Vitamin D primarily regulates calcium metabolism by determining the movement of calcium from intestines to blood and from blood to bone. It interacts with parathyroid hormone and calcitonin (see hormone, animal) in controlling calcium levels. Thus vitamin D is today more legitimately considered a hormone rather than a vitamin.

Vitamin E is considered to have possible value in decreasing the risk of cancer; it has shown little therapeutic value in other diseases. Fortunately, it is relatively nontoxic. Vitamin K is essential for synthesis by the liver of several factors necessary for the clotting of blood. A wide variety of vegetables, egg yolk, liver, and fish oils contain this vitamin.

With the exception of vitamin C (ascorbic acid), water-soluble vitamins belong mainly to what has been termed the B complex of vitamins. The better-known B vitamins are thiamine (B(1)), riboflavin (B(2)), niacin (B(3)), pyridoxine (B(6)), pantothenic acid, lecithin, choline, inositol, and paraaminobenzoic acid (PABA). Two other members are folic acid and cyanocobalamin (B(12)). Yeast and liver are natural sources of most of these vitamins.

Thiamine, the first B vitamin functions as a coenzyme in the form of thiamine pyrophosphate and is important in carbohydrate intermediary metabolism.

Riboflavin (B(2) serves as coenzymes for a wide variety of respiratory proteins (see metabolism).

Vitamin B(6), functions in human metabolism in the conversion processes of amino acids, including decarboxylation, transamination, and racemization.

In the body folic acid is converted to folinic acid (5-formyl-tetrahydro-folic acid), the coenzyme form, which accepts 1-carbon units important in the metabolism of many body compounds. Nucleic acid synthesis cannot take place without the presence of folic acid.

Vitamin B(12), almost all organisms need this vitamin but only in very small amounts.

For vitamin C, a sufficient daily intake of fresh orange juice provides enough of the vitamin for most purposes. The body's requirements for calcium are generally met by eating or drinking dairy products, especially milk. Most calcium (90 percent) is stored in bone, with a constant exchange occurring among blood, tissue, and bone.

Iron is a vital component of hemoglobin and also of certain respiratory enzymes. Foods high in iron content include meat (liver and heart), egg yolk, wheat germ, and most green vegetables. The average diet contains 10 to 15 mg a day, adequate for most people.

Magnesium is an essential element in human metabolism and functions in the activities of muscles and nerves, protein synthesis, and many other reactions. Fluorine as fluoride is a requirement to bind calcium in bones. Micro amounts of such elements as boron, chromium, chlorine, copper, manganese, molybdenum, selenium, silicon, sulfur, and vanadium are considered necessary to health.

Normal diets appear to provide adequate amounts of trace minerals, but effects such as the linking of high levels of fructose in the diet with copper-deficiency problems are the subject of ongoing research. Vitamins and minerals are an important factor to keeping yourself healthy.

When I started incorporating vitamins into my daily schedule, I began noticing a change in the way I felt physically. When I started eating healthily, I started using a variety of vitamins and herbs that were suppose to be helpful for epilepsy disorders. The vitamins I used were L-Taurine L-tyrosine(amino acids), vitamin B6 and B12, calcium and folic acid. They called a herb that I also had tried a black cohosh. Black cohosh is an eastern North American perennial herb Cimicifuga racemosa. It has a powerful action as a relaxant and a normalizer of the female reproductive system. It may be used in cases of painful or delayed menstruation, ovarian cramps or cramping pain in the womb. It has a normalizing action on the balance of female sex hormones and may be used safely to regain normal hormonal activity. It is used often for the treatment of neurological pain. As a relaxing nervine it may be used in many situations where such a agent is needed.

Medical research has not proven that these vitamins and herbs stop seizures. Nevertheless, they have been used for decades and said to be beneficial. I still have the same amount of seizures (two to three a month), but I have noticed an increase in my energy. I also had a couple of incidents when I was about to go into an aura. For the first time, I could work with my body and stop myself from having an aura or petite mal seizure by using relaxation exercises. I took deep breaths and slowly released the air through my mouth as I thought positive thoughts.

I have recently incorporated an extra iron vitamin into my diet. Remember, if you decide to use vitamins as a part of your daily diet than it is always safe to first discuss it with your doctor.

I believe exercise can help control seizures. Epilepsy does not stop you from being athletic and keeping your body in shape. Some of the greatest athletes had epilepsy. French cyclist Marion Clignet won a silver medal in the 1996 Olympics. Hal Lanier, a former shortstop with the San Francisco Giant; Greg Walker, a former first baseman with the Chicago White Sox, and Buddy Bell, who played seventeen seasons of professional baseball before retiring in 1988, all reportedly had epilepsy as did basketball player Bobby Jones, who played for the Denver Nuggets and Philadelphia '76ers. Exercise helps to build or maintain strength and endurance and to make the body healthier. Exercising is good because it also helps you spiritually. Exercise has both physical and psychological benefits. Regular exercise helps develop muscle tone and strength and control weight. Besides strengthening the muscles, including the heart, regular exercise is believed to make bones stronger by increasing calcium uptake.

Exercise would be extremely beneficial for all individuals, especially for epileptics' who have been using Tegretol for many years. The main problems associated with Tegretol are that it causes your bones to ache. Exercise reduces high blood pressure and cholesterol levels.

Psychologically, regular exercise contributes to a feeling of well-being, and relieves stress. It helps you to feel at peace with yourself. In a study reported in the professional journal Epilepsia, conducted at the department of psychology, University of Alabama at Birmingham exercise proved to have a positive effect on the lives of a hundred and thirty-three people with epilepsy. Fifty-four of them were men and seventy-nine of them were women. Those who exercise intensely at least three times a week for a minimum of twenty minutes reported fewer problems with depression and stress.

Another study was also done on how exercise effects epileptics was done at the University of sport and Physical Education. In this study fifteen Norwegian women with drug-resistant epilepsy spent fifteen weeks taking exercise classes twice a week for an hour. They combined aerobic dancing with strength training and stretching. The median number of seizures decreased from 2.9 to 1.7 during the experimental exercise phase. The women also had fewer health complaints, such as muscle pains, sleep problems and fatigue.

People who exercise are regularly more likely to continue exercise throughout their lives. Once I got into the habit of exercising, it no longer became a chore. Exercising became a physical activity that I enjoyed doing in my spare time. I made sure that I scheduled my days so I would at least have three to four days of exercise. Exercising should take place at least every other day foe a period of fifteen to sixty minutes.

I enjoy walking, floor aerobics, weights and working on the machines. I would work out a little each day and exercise with the TV or the radio. Whatever motivated me then, but remember before you begin any exercise program you should check with your doctor first.

When I exercised it made me feel good inside. Exercise should be some activity that you can do that will not strain your body. It can be walking, jogging, running, aerobics, bench stepping, hiking, jazzercize, body building, swimming, dance or anything that you enjoy. You should do some kind of exercise to keep your body in shape. The older you become the more important is to exercise. Exercise affects the aging body, helping to maintain fitness and slow down the physical effects of aging. If not properly exercised, the aging body can develop problems in the muscles, bones and cardiovascular system. As you get older your muscles begin to wither away and lose their tone, leading to more frequent tearing of the tendons in the muscles. Your bones become weak and brittle, fracturing easily and more often. So it is important that you take responsibility and keep yourself in good shape. Keeping yourself healthy will help you and your epilepsy.

KEEPING YOURSELF IN SPIRITUAL AND EMOTIONAL GOOD HEALTH:

As I was working to accept my epilepsy, I noticed myself changing emotionally. I felt better about myself. I would look in the mirror and be proud of the person I was seeing.

I remember in college my marketing professor assigned us a book to read. It was the most boring book I ever read in my life. I could feel the stress increase as I kept reading the book. The book had no purpose and I could not understand why he would assign us to read this book. Suddenly I felt an aura start to come on and then the rest of the seizure. My point is that I could have avoided the stress by putting the book the down and reading it at different times. I had created the stress myself. We have the power to control stress and thus help our body avoid seizures. We need to understand how our bodies work and listen to its messages. Because we have epilepsy, we need to be a little more careful than the average individual.

I never thought when I was growing up as a child that I would have to be limited in enjoying certain activities I wanted to explore. I thought I could do everything. I realize now, as a young woman, there is no reason for me to lower my expectations, but there is also no reason to push myself over the limit. No one on this earth is a 100% perfect. We all have our faults. I work all the time by trying to make myself into a stronger human being emotionally, physically and spiritually. Working on myself makes me feel like I can fight the battle of epilepsy and so can you! Everybody has different characteristics that make up their personalities. Epilepsy is just one part of me. I cannot change the fact that I am epileptic. I have to just accept it the fact that I have epilepsy and learn to live with it productively. You will succeed and become a better person, if you think positively and productively. You will feel the strength in yourself to accept your epilepsy. Think about who you and where you are headed in life. It is up to you to make something of yourself.

Here is exercises to help you improve yourself physically mentally and spiritually. I call this the spirituality builder.   It uses all your muscles and is designed to help you develop strength and flexibility in the body, increasing circulation, and stretching. These exercises will help you feel good and at peace with yourself. I do these exercises frequently. It helped me feel like I had full control with myself. We may not have control over ourselves when we have seizures; however, we do have the power to figure out how to deal with our epilepsy so it does not become a problem in our lives.

THE EXERCISE
1. Lie on your back with your arms at your sides. Adjust your body to a comfortable position.
2. Slowly relaxing all your muscles in your body starting with the feet and then working your way up to your head.

3. Keep your eyes closed, concentrating on what you see inside yourself. Focus on what you feel and what you want to feel like.
4. Slowly raise your body upright, bending forward
5. Then bend to your right side
6. Then to your left side
7. Then back to step one position
8. Remember to take deep breaths during this exercise and breathe slowly.
9. Do this for a minimum of fifteen minutes a day.

EXERCISE TWO

This exercise should be done twice a day for 5-15 minutes in a quiet room free from disturbance.

1. Rest on your back with head and neck comfortably supported
2. Rest hands on upper abdomen, close your eyes and settle in a comfortable position.
3. Breathe slowly, deeply and rhythmically. Inhalation should be slow, unforced and unhurried. Silently count to 4, 5 or 6, whatever feels right for you.
4. When inhalation is complete, slowly inhale through the nose. Count this breathing out, as when breathing in. The exhalation should take as long as the inhalation. There should be no sense of strain. If initially you feel you have breathed your fullest at a count of three, that is alright. Try gradually to slow down the rhythm until a slow count of 5 or 6 is possible, with a pause of 2 or 3 between in and out breathing.
5. This pattern of breathing should be repeated 15 or 20 times and since each cycle should take about 15 seconds, this exercise should take about 5 minutes to do.
6. Once the mechanics of this exercise have been mastered, try to introduce thoughts at different parts of the cycle. On inhalation try to sense a feeling of warmth and energy entering the body with the air. On exhalation sense a feeling of sinking and settling deeper into the surface you are lying on.

7. On completion do not get up immediately but rest for a minute or two, allowing the mind to become aware of any sensations or stillness, warmth, heaviness etc. Once mastered, this exercise can be used to help you cope with any situation, so you don't become over agitated.

EXERCISE THREE

Often tension is focused in the muscles of the body itself, and the following exercise itself can release such tightness and allow the mind to be at ease. It is best to begin this exercise with a few cycles of deep breathing.

1. Lie down or sit down in a reclining chair.
2. Avoid distractions and wear clothes that are comfortable.
3. Starting with the feet, try to feel or sense that the muscles of the area are not actively tense.
4. Then deliberately tighten the muscles, curling the toes under and holding the tension for 5 or 10 seconds.
5. Then tense them even more strongly for a few more seconds before letting go of all the tension and sensing the feeling of release.
6. Try to consciously understand what this feels like, especially in comparison with the tense state in which they were held.
7. Exercise the calf muscles in the same way. First sense the state the muscles are in, then tense them, hold them in position, and then tense them even more before letting go. Positively sense of relief. If cramping occurs, stop tensing that area immediately and go on to the next area.
8. After the calf go on to exercising the knees, then the upper leg, thighs, buttocks, back, abdomen, chest, shoulders, arms, hands, neck, head and face. The particular order is irrelevant, as long as these areas are exercised the same way.
9. Some areas may need extra attention. For example, in the abdomen the tensing of the muscle can be achieved either by contracting (pulling in the tummy) or by stretching (pushing outwards). This variation in tensing is suitable to many muscles in the body.

10. There are between 20 and 25 of these areas depending how you go about it. Give each about 5-10 seconds of tensing and another 5-10 seconds of letting go. It should take 8-10 minutes to complete this exercise. After the exercise, try to relax for a couple of minutes.

11. Focus the mind on the whole body. Sense it as heavy and content, free of tension. You can do this by doing a few cycles of deep breathing.

SECTION FOUR

ABOUT THE AUTHOR

Chapter 11

ABOUT THE AUTHOR

I got epilepsy at the age of five. I had contracted a sore throat and an ear infection. My mother had brought me to the doctor's office that evening and the pediatrician had put me on penicillin and told my mother to have me rest in bed. No one thought much of it at the time. When one is young, your immune system is weak and catching any bug surfacing in the air is all too easy. Especially, sore throats and ear infections, the most common sicknesses afflicting young children.

I rested in bed and I was on the penicillin for about ten days. My mother recalls that on the tenth night when she put me to bed, my lips were more red than usual. The next morning about 8:00 A.M., my mother woke up because she heard unusual noises coming from my room that sounded like I was choking on my saliva. She found me in my bed turning blue and having a convulsion. This was the first time I ever had a seizure.

She ran to the phone to call the ambulance and had me rushed to the hospital. They brought me to the emergency room and hurried me to the isolation ward. They had no idea if the seizure was brought on by any type of serious or contagious illness. The doctors at the hospital diagnosed the convulsion as a grand mal seizure, a We also know this type of seizure as generalized tonic clonic seizure.

I fell to the floor, my eyes rolled to the left and my whole body began to shake. My teeth began to chatter, and I started to foam at the mouth and choke on my saliva and my skin color began to turn bluish because of the lack of oxygen I was enduring. All I remember is waking up in a hospital bed. My parents were in the room with me.

They administered many tests to try to diagnose the cause of the grand mal seizure. The doctors finally concluded that the grand mal seizure came from a virus. The virus I had was not an ordinary virus. It was a virus known as encephalitis. The doctors had told my parents that the bacteria from the ear infection had traveled to my head and that the virus was still in my brain. Doctors had told my parents that the viral encephalitis had to leave my brain naturally on its own. Doctors were not sure when the germ would leave my brain. Then said that while the virus was in my brain that it could possibly leave me with some type of brain damage. I was in an induced coma for four days after the grand mal seizure. The doctor had told my parents while I was in a coma that if I were to come out alive I would probably have severe brain damage or I could become paralyzed in a wheel chair.

This horrible news devastated my parents, but they never gave up hope. On the fourth day while I was in a coma, my father lay by my bedside and began praying to a saint. My parents told me years later that after my dad finished praying a tear drop rolled off from my eye and down my face and I woke up. They tested me right away and found that the infection had traveled to my brain and caused left-sided scare tissue damage. The doctor told my parents I was very fortunate; then had expected the outcome to be much worse. Which was the reason for me developing epilepsy.

The scar tissue damage I generated is very small and does not interfere with the way I think or function. The only problem that developed was that I found some difficulties with my long-term memory and I have trouble with my usage of words occasionally. When I am talking, I have problems remembering the word I want to use. So instead, I need to compensate with another word. This could be because the part of the brain that controls vocabulary is right next to the memory. The scar tissue damage is probably between both areas, I am assuming. These two functions of the brain are close to one another, This is probably the reason I have difficulties with both areas. This is a very minor handicap compared to other cases of epilepsy that were brought to my attention. I am very lucky. God was definitely watching over me.

Phenobarbital controlled my seizures, until the age of nine. Before I was nine, the only time I would experience a seizure was when I had an high fever. When I had a high temperature, I usually would have a grand-mal seizure. Phenobarbital is known today to be a barbiturate and is not used as frequently on epileptic patients.

At nine, my body began to go through the stages of womanhood. This is when I experienced puberty. Once my hormones started changing I began developing more seizures. My seizures would occur around the time of menstruation and ovulation. My neurologist told me that I was retaining water on my brain during this time of the month.

My aura's begin with a feeling of fear or paranoia. When I have a aura I start to feel scared and begin to think that someone or something is going to hurt me. For instance, if I were in a car while a seizure was beginning to occur, and we were driving where there were a lot of trees, I would begin to feel like someone was going to pop out from the trees and hurt me physically. After encountering that scared feeling, I would then start to feel 'a tingling feeling in my feet.' The tingling sensation would develop into a feeling of being electrocuted, as if one put your finger in an electrical socket. The electrical sensation would travel up my leg to my head. Once the current of electricity reached my brain the aura would then end and I would lose consciousness.

When I endured a seizure, my eyes would roll to the left, my hands would move toward the left side also, my teeth would chatter and my mouth would foam with saliva. My seizures would occur almost any time of the day. My seizures mostly lasted for about thirty to forty-five seconds. Then I would come out of the seizures sometimes with memory loss depending how severe the seizure was then. I would also feel fatigue after a seizure and would usually have take a nap. My seizures were continuing to occur more frequently as I got older, so my neurologist felt that the medication Phenobarbital was no longer controlling my seizures. The neurologists wanted to administer another medicine combined with Phenobarbital to try to stop my seizures from occurring.

When I turned twelve, they put me on another drug called Tegretol. The neurologists were hoping that the combination of the Phenobarbital and Tegretol would help regulate my seizures. I always kept a positive out-look, hoping this would be the medicine that would completely control my seizures. My body seemed to agree with this medicine. The combination of both drugs worked well in my body. My seizures were decreasing monthly. Unfortunately, I was taking large doses of both medications.

At the age of eighteen, my seizures were well under control and my neurologist gave me permission to drive a car feeling that my safety was no longer in jeopardy or that could endanger someone's life while driving. I was so excited.

Unfortunately, after a few years, I had to stop driving because my seizures began to increase to two or three a month. The seizures occurred mainly at the time my hormones were changing during ovulation or menstruation, so I had to be always on guard. My seizures would occur four to five days before or after ovulation and menstruation. I was capable of having a seizure at anytime of the month.

I was not going to let the fact that I could not drive discourage me. I came to the conclusion that one needs to work with what one has and make the best of it. I was going to focus on just the positive aspects of my life and not let epilepsy get me down. I refused to let epilepsy depress or control me. If Vincent Van Gogh could be a famous painter despite being epileptic, then I should be able to become something good in life too. I believe God does everything for a reason. We need to look at life on a positive note. My friends and family have been extremely supportive and willing to help me in any way they can. My family and friends are always willing to drive me anywhere I need to go. If they saw that I was struggling and having a hard time dealing with my epilepsy for whatever reason they always offered their support and love. They understand that sometimes it can become stressful or frustrating when one wants to go somewhere and one has to rely on others to get to the there.

I feel uncomfortable sometimes asking people for car rides because I know everyone has their own lives to live and responsibilities that they need to attend to. I do not want others to feel obligated to take me places when I have to go somewhere but, I have gotten better when it comes to reaching out to others for help, though I have always been a self-reliant person. When one has epilepsy, one needs to realize that you cannot do everything by yourself. Having seizures does create problems, but it does not stop us from reaching our destinations. In order for us to do everything we want too, we need to realize that we have to reach out for other people's support and love. Having other people's love and support is a necessity in life. No one can make it through this life alone. My family and friends have helped make my life a lot less stressful. Dealing with epilepsy for once had become a easier and a more pleasant experience.

In my twenties, my neurologist and I decided to stop the Phenobarbital. I chose to stop the phenobarbital because my seizures were still persisting and were not decreasing. New drugs came on the market for epilepsy and were working well with other people who had the disorder. Also, they knew the newer drugs on the market to be healthier and safer to use.

I eagerly wanted to stop having seizures completely, so I decided to try a few new medications. If worse came to worst, I could always go back onto my original medication. I tried Depakote, Felbatol, Dilantin and Nervone with the Tegretol, yet nothing seemed to stop the seizures from coming.

My neurologist began to try to encourage me to go for temporal brain surgery. My family and friends gave me much support while I was making one of the most important decisions of my life. Surgery may be an option if a tumor is causing the epilepsy in the brain, or if the medication fails to control the seizures. Surgery usually becomes an option when the seizures begin in one small area of the brain. If such an area can be found, the surgeon will remove it, and usually the seizures will then stop, or reduce, but they will only operate when the possible benefits outweigh the risks.

I was so terrified when my doctor had suggested that I should go for testing to see if I were a candidate for brain surgery. Every time he mentioned that I go for brain surgery I would ignore his comment and discuss the new medicines on the market for seizure control. I was terrified of the thought of brain surgery. My neurologist gave me phone numbers of other individuals with epilepsy who went through the surgery and had wonderful success. The names and numbers of the people he gave me had stopped taking seizures either completely or barely ever would have a seizure after having the surgery. One person whom I spoke to gave me detailed descriptions of what to expect. She helped motivate me and feel relaxed. The young woman I spoke with was enthusiastic about the surgical procedure that my neurologist wanted me to undergo. After the surgery, she would have seizures infrequently instead of constantly. Life became so much easier for her once her seizures decreased to the point where she was almost seizure free.

At age twenty-two, in January of 1995, I finally decided to go for testing. I traveled to Chicago with my fiancee and father to Rush-Presbyterian St. Lukes Medical Center to have the doctors specializing in an epileptic surgery; test me. According to statistics, of the 150,000 people with epilepsy who are candidates for surgery, only about 1,000 a year have it done. To be a candidate for surgery, they must trace the seizures to one small area of damaged brain tissue and they cannot control them with medication. Before pre-surgical evaluation is completed, anti-epileptic drug treatments are fully explored Statistics also show that medication does not work for at least a third of those who have the disorder.

They scheduled me for diagnostic work up at the hospital. Upon admission, they took me to my room where they gave blood tests and hooked me to an EEG for continuous twenty-four hour (EEG) monitoring. They monitor the 24-hours-a-day EEG on an audio-video. A team of registered EEG technologists and electrical engineers that maintain the recording equipment. Electrodes always remain attached, but the patient is free to move around the room. They may monitor the patient up to two or three weeks before desired results are conclusive.

One of the doctor's goals is to find the exact location of the scar tissue damage and the depth of the scar tissue. To do this they gave me a test called the magnetic resonance imaging (MRI). Neuropsychological tests were also done. These are IQ, memory and speech tests. These tell the doctors more about where the seizures, (or the brain damage, that is causing the seizures), are found. They administered many other tests to see if I were a qualified patient for epileptic brain surgery.

My fiancee and father were great support. They stood by my side day and night. The emotional stress of the tests and thinking that it was a possibility that I could be going through the surgery made me feel terrified.

Having my fiancee and father there released so much anxiety and made the whole time at the hospital easier.

The neurologist was unable to tell if the seizures were coming from left frontal or the left temporal part of the brain. The next test scheduled was minor surgery to evaluate where the scar tissue was found. The anesthesiologist came in to give me an anaesthetic and inserted a little too much into my face. My one side of my face became numb and stopped functioning. It was not a big deal. Nevertheless, I became frantic and told my fiancee and father that I had enough and wanted to go home. I was young at the time and the whole surgery notion was very hard for me to handle. I was not strong enough emotionally to go through brain surgery. When that incident happened I kept thinking to myself what if something happens to me while I am in surgery. What if they make a mistake? I am so young and I have a whole life ahead of me. Maybe I should be appreciative and be happy with the things God has given me. No matter how easy my fiancee and father made it for me by being there, I could not go undergo anymore testing or surgery. I decided to fly back home the next day.

For me brain surgery was not the answer, but for some it is the solution. Cindy, a wonderful young woman who has shared her epileptic experiences with me has given some valuable information on brain surgery.

In a study, of eighty-nine patients with medically refractory epilepsy whom they consecutively treated with anterior temporal lobectomy between 1986 and 1990. Dr. Michael R Sperling, reports in the Journal of the American Medical Association (470), that "five years after surgery, of sixty-two patients, followed, 70% were seizure-free, 9% had seizures on fewer than three days per year or exclusively had nocturnal seizures, 11% greater than 8% reduction in seizure frequency and 4% died of causes unrelated to the surgery.

If one were to ask these people how they feel, most likely they will say, "never better!" If one asks them if they would go through the surgery again, they will say without a doubt, Yes, they would! To meet these people, to see them, to talk to with them, one would never know what they have been through.

When I came home from Chicago, I scheduled an appointment to go see my neurologist. My doctor put me in two research medicine programs. I was about 85% seizure-free at this time. I was in college at this time, I figured this would probably be the best time to participate in new lab research study programs. I would try any new epileptic medicines that the FDA in the United States has not approved for commercial use and maybe I would get lucky. If these medicines had a positive effect and helped control my seizures then they would sponsor the medication after the study. If nothing good comes out of the lab research programs; this would be the time to start experimenting with new medicines that recently came on the market. I wanted to participate in the research study also because I had tried every medicine on the market and none of them had helped me become seizure free.

One research study I took part in was for Tiagabine H.L. Three hundred patients with partial seizures will took part in this nationwide study. The research study took seven months to complete. The research study was a two-part analysis. They called the one part of the study the baseline phase. This is where one goes for tests to master your level of intelligence and see where your strengths and weaknesses lied.

While I was in this study, they required me to see a neurologist twice a week for examinations and blood tests. I had to keep track of all my seizures by using calendars developed by the study. The calendars would keep track of my seizures to see when I was taking them and the type of seizures I was experiencing. The study consisted of two unrelated types of medicines;

Tiagabine and Dilantin. They called this portion of the study the double blind phase. One had no idea what medicine they were going to receive. You received either Tiagabine H.L. or Dilantine. If they gave them Dilantin and the medicine fails, then they would slowly wean the individual off the drug and put them on Tiagabine(which was the experimental drug).

The first medication they put me on was Dilantine. I had developed a strong reaction to the drug. For the first few days, I felt fine on the medication; however, once the medicine began to circulate in my blood stream, I then developed a fever and a horrible skin rash from head to toe. I started to develop cold sores around my mouth and on my tongue. The sores were exceedingly painful. It was so painful that I was unable to eat anything for a week or so. The only thing I could put in my system was water. They put me in bed rest for a couple of weeks. I lost much weight during this time because I was not eating anything.

When they put me on the Tiagabine I felt optimistic that my seizures were going to get better. My complex partial seizures lessened to focal seizures. I was hoping that the intensity of the seizures would keep decreasing till I became seizure-free on the medicine. During this time the seizures were so slight I was not even experiencing any memory loss after a seizure or feeling fatigue after encountering a seizure, two side effects I struggled with ever since I developed epilepsy. My memory began to feel sharper and I felt much more energetic. The emotional frustration and pain of having a seizure started decreased and I was finally better able to cope with my epilepsy. My only problem was that my seizure were still occurring two to three times a month.

I decided to try another new medicine that came on the market. I did not want to have even two to three seizures a month, though my side effects from the seizures went away. The reason I started to try all these medicines in the first place was to find a drug that would control my seizures 100 percent. I was very eager to try to find a medicine that would control my seizures. They called the medicine I was about to start Tegretol RX. When I was on Tegretol I seemed to respond well to the medicine. The only side effect I had on this medicine was that I felt a little tired on Tegretol. I had not experienced any other side effects and the medicine controlled my seizures 90 percent. Tegretol RX was exactly like Tegretol except that it is supposed to stay longer in your blood stream.

My neurologist thought that this medicine would be a good medicine to try. He weaned me off the Phenobarbital I was currently taking at the time and put me on just Tegretol RX with a water pill called Diamox at 250mg.

Diamox is a water pill that relieves fluid from the brain. My neurologist had instructed me to take Diamox four days before and after my ovulation. He also had me take Diamox four days before and after my menstruation process. This is the time when I would accumulate water on my brain, which caused pressure that would cause the seizures to occur.

At twenty-five, Tegretol RX, Diamox and the small dosage of Phenobarbital were controlling my seizures the same as the Tegretol and Phenobarbital which I was using before. My neurologist had mentioned to me that I should not get discouraged.

These drugs were not good for your body. Phenobarbital is not good because it is a barbiturate. Tegretol is not good because it eats away the liver, muscle and bones. It takes a long time for the side effects of Tegretol to start, but eventually it will in effect major parts of your body. I was worried because I started to use Tegretol at the age of nine, it has only been recently since I started to experiment with other drugs. Tegretol helped me the best out to which out of all the other medications, but it did not fully control my seizures.

My neurologist had another research drug that came out that he had access. He suggested that I participate in the study lab research program for Oxcarbazepine, a new medicine that had many positive responses among epileptics in Europe. This study program is similar to the one I mentioned earlier. When they put me on this medicine, I was not 100% seizure free and I still had an average of three complex partial seizures a month. Although I liked this medication better than the Tiagabine. I was feeling even more energetic with the Oxcarbazepine. When they were administering me all the other medications, I had almost the same degree of stamina. The Tegretol RX, I tried right before this made me feel the most lackadaisical. I was constantly taking naps. On this medication I felt no need to have to stop what I was doing because of fatigue. My memory is even sharper on Oxcarbazepine than the Tiagabine. I can respond quicker to things. I feel alive and for the first time in a long time. I can appreciate life and enjoy the wonderful things that life has blessed me with. I have a deep sense of care inside myself and I had not felt this way in a long time. I decided that although I am still having seizures, I am not going to stop this medicine. The few seizures I have are worth it, if I feel this wonderful.

When I told my neurologist how I was feeling and the few seizures I was still having monthly he decided to try to combine the Oxcarbazepine with another medication. He wanted to see if two anti-epileptic drugs would control my seizures better.

They called the first medicine my neurologist used Topamax. They gave me 25rng. This medicine did not agree well with my body. The medicine made me feel really tired. All I wanted to do was sleep. This medicine made me feel most fatigued from all the medicines I have attempted in the past. My thinking capacity became much slower and my speech became a little slurred. I was unable to function at work or anywhere for that matter. I was constantly in a daze and felt horrible. There was no way I could have gone through the rest of my life feeling this way. I was in my own little world, unable to enjoy the life that God gave me. Although I was feeling this way, I still felt it was only fair to give my body time to adjust to the medicine. I thought if I gave the medicine time the side effects would eventually wear off, so I could function better. Six weeks later, I was still having the same side effects. Emotionally, I was not able to continue feeling this way. I spoke to my neurologist and he had me weaned off the Topamax and used Phenobarbital as a second medicine. This combination worked wonderfully. I was still having seizures, yet the intensity of the seizure was decreasing.

It may sound like I have everything under control. It may also sound like epilepsy has not affected my life. But I will be honest with you, it has been hard to learn to live with epilepsy. I have had my highs and lows. Epilepsy has made me feel depressed at times and has gotten me down. Sometimes, having epilepsy has made me feel like an outcast. I have realized in the past couple years that you can do anything they want in life, if you try hard enough and put your mind to it. You need to understand that you can become your worst enemy if you let yourself. **YOU CANNOT GIVE UP.** You need to keep trying until you succeed. Very rarely does anything come easy. The percentage of people that are seizure-free from medications is not that high. Although, there are people out there who are seizure-free due to anti-epileptic medications on the market and this is what we need to focus on. It has been tough for me with all the testing and medical let downs, but I focus on the positive and try to avoid the negative. I have grown as a person from all these experiences both mentally and spiritually.

Mentally it has helped me mature and accept myself for whom I am. Accepting yourself is one of the most important steps to healing. You need to understand that yes, and I am epileptic and nothing going to change the fact that I am. Yes, I may find a drug that controls my seizures, but that does not change the fact that I am epileptic.

Spiritually I have learned a lot about myself; I learned what my wants and what my needs are. I have also learned that one cannot let having epilepsy control their life. Yes, I have epilepsy, but I do not have to stop living. Life goes on! One needs to be proud of who they are.

I am determined to live a normal life. You cannot compare your life to someone else's life. If you do that you're going to be unhappy. You need to love yourself and be satisfied with the life you lead and if you're not satisfied than change it! You need to realize also that there are plenty of people who take medicine and many individuals do not drive for lots of other reasons. You should not feel ashamed or feel different from others. We all have a special beauty within us. No one is perfect or has a life that is flawless.

So if you have epilepsy do not, be ashamed that you are epileptic. Someone that I met a while back taught me that there is nothing wrong with having epilepsy. Throughout the book, I have letters of people telling their experiences of living with epilepsy and how they feel having the disorder. I learned so many valuable things from all the letters I have received. It is very easy to begin to feel sorry for yourself until you realize that some people may have it a lot worse. It has also helped me feel better to know that there are many other epileptics in this world. We may have different seizures, but our feelings about living with epilepsy are all very similar.

I truly believe that all things happen for a reason. I believe that our lives are planned for us a head of time. There is nothing wrong with having epilepsy. Epilepsy is something that you should not be ashamed of or hide. Having epilepsy has taught me to appreciate life and appreciate what God has given me. It has helped me develop confidence in myself and to love myself for who I am. Epilepsy has also made me want to reach out and help others.

Chapter 12

HAVING A BABY WITH EPILEPSY

Did you know that women with epilepsy have fewer children than any other women? This could be because of personal choice, but research has indicated that women with epilepsy have a higher rate of menstrual cycle irregularities and other gynecological problems that may interfere with fertility.

Ever since I was a little girl playing with dolls in my playroom, I always dreamed of having a baby and becoming a mother. I always wanted a family of my own that I could take care of. I remember when I was young my mother tried to explain to me that because I took medicine because I had seizures, there was a possibility that I might not be able to have children. She told me that I might have to adopt and that you could love someone as your own although they did not come from you biologically. Despite her warning, I was not going to let having epilepsy stop me from having a beautiful child. I felt no different from anyone on this planet.

I knew deep down inside that someday I was going to be a wife and a mother to my own wonderful family. In October of 1997, I became pregnant with my first child. My husband and I were thrilled, but we were also scared. Like all parents we were hoping and praying for a healthy child, and were afraid that the medications I was taking would do to harm the baby. I was a little nervous during the pregnancy, but something inside told me that everything was going to be all right. I was no longer afraid, and became more excited than ever.

Having your first child brings out many fears because you do not know what to expect and is going to happen. Women with epilepsy do have a greater risk of having a baby with certain kinds of birth defects. The rate is 4—6% for women with epilepsy, compared with the rate of 2—3% in the general population.

In the past, they discouraged women with epilepsy from having children and sometimes were sterilized against their will to prevent pregnancy. However, now the public's understanding of epilepsy has grown, and the medical community has useful information to share with women who have seizures and want to become pregnant. More than 90% of women with epilepsy who choose to become pregnant have healthy babies.

When I told my neurologist that I was pregnant he was optimistic. He explained to me that there was special concerns I had to consider. One of his main concerns was the fact that I was taking Phenobarbital. Although I was consuming a small dosage, he still was worried. If he knew six months in advance before I got pregnant, he would have taken me off the Phenobarbital. Personally, I am happy that I was on the medicine during my pregnancy. Phenobarbital always seemed to control my seizures well when combined with the appropriate medication. I was afraid if I did not have the Phenobarbital in my system that my seizures would worsen and would harm to the baby. Every time you have a seizure while you are pregnant you cause oxygen deficiency for the baby. Also if I fell during a seizure, for example, off the bed I could hurt the baby.

I was very careful during my pregnancy. I went to every appointment I had with my neurologist and OB-GYN. I continuously had an EEG done to make sure everything was all right. I took folic acid vitamins on a daily basis.

I was blessed. It was a very easy pregnancy. I had not experienced any morning sickness and felt energetic and happy. I was lucky because women with epilepsy are more likely to have morning sickness and vaginal bleeding. I had neither during my pregnancy.

Every morning I ate an egg for protein. I drank plenty of milk for the calcium and orange juice for the vitamin C. I ate meat and some pasta and was constantly eating vegetables. I broke everything up into equal shares, so I would not give myself too much of one type of food and protein.

As time went on my appetite began to increase and I started to become increasingly tired. I was having no problems with the medicine I was taking; the only problem I encountered during the pregnancy was that when I entered this research program. I had signed a prodical stating that I would not get pregnant during the study. When the hospital had found out about my pregnancy, they wanted to stop me using Oxicarbazepine immediately (the research drug). The hospital and pharmaceutical company sponsoring the study did not want to take any responsibility God forbid something happened to the baby do to the research drug.

I was upset because, as I had mentioned earlier this medication had made dramatic changes in my life for the better. They stated that this drug did well in Europe for women who were pregnant and had epilepsy. I felt it would be unhealthy for the baby just to take me off the medicine and put me on a new drug. There were not many drugs on the market that will control my seizures and help me to function normally. I wanted to be able to be a good mother, but how could I do that if my seizures were uncontrolled and my mind unstable because of the medication. The only drug that could help my seizures was not healthy for myself or for the baby. That medicine was Tegretol. Eventually we convinced the research committee and hospital to let me use the research medicine during my pregnancy. My neurologist fought vigorously to keep me on the medicine, and with his help and our determination I was able to.

Ever since I became pregnant, my seizures have been only occurring in my sleep. My seizures are usually focal or complex partial and last about thirty to forty-five seconds. I have been very happy that I have been only experiencing seizures in my sleep. Having the seizures in my sleep right next to my husband made me feel safer because he was able to see the seizure and he was able to help me if I needed it.

My pregnancy was pleasureful. In the second part of my pregnancy about in my fourth month I went for a second level sonagram. This son-agram was more sophisticated and could detect many more signs of a birth defect. Everything came out normal. This released so much tension and put our hearts at ease in the 6th month, I went for another sonagram. I did not have to go, but my husband and I just wanted to hear the doctors say that everything was all right, which they did.

Every day I was experiencing something new. Either my stomach was stretching or I wake up to find my stomach leaning toward the left and the next day it would be leaning toward the right. I remember the first time the baby kicked me. It was such an exciting experience to feel a living, breathing body inside yourself move.

I worked until my seventh month. When I got into my seventh month I began to feel increasingly tired and my energy level was quickly dropping. I no longer was able to work a seven-hour day, so I took a maternity leave of absence and rested at home.

In my eighth month I went through one standard sonagram. The sonagram came out normal.

My whole pregnancy was wonderful. I did not experience any nausea or morning sickness. I had no complications and everything went smoothly.

I was going to the neurologist more frequently. They had me to get EEG's done on a more regular basis to keep track of my progress. The reason for this is that, though women with epilepsy have the same risks as women who do not have epilepsy, "a woman who is taking anti-epileptic medicines needs to be under careful attention before getting pregnant, during pregnancy and delivery, and even in the first six to twelve weeks after delivery, "said Robert J. Gumnit, MD, a clinical professor of neurology and neurosurgery at the University of Minnesota. However, if you're planning a family or in the midst of a pregnancy and have epilepsy, don't let your worry feelings consume your life. "More than 90% of the time, everything goes well without difficulties," reported Dr. Gumnit.

I was excited about having the baby. Deep down inside my heart I knew the baby would be healthy and beautiful. Something inside me has already told me not to worry. Of course, one loves what God gives them and I truly believe that God does not dish out anything one cannot handle.

I gave birth to my baby eight months and two weeks into the pregnancy. The baby began kicking more than usual. The last two nights before I went into labor, the baby had kicked me sixty times one night and one hundred and thirty times the other night. The second night, I went to bed and I had a grand-mal seizure. I had not had a grand-mal seizure in such a long time. In my whole lifetime I may have had a total of five grand-mal seizures. I did not even recognize that I had one. If my husband had not told me the next morning, I would have never of known.

When I told my neurologist he was very worried and he wanted me to get induced and have the baby right away. He was afraid I would take more seizures as critical and this would cause the baby to get hurt. We took his advice and went to the hospital to get induced. They checked me in and did the necessary procedures. I had contractions for fourteen hours and kept calling the nurse in, telling her it's time. What I thought were the major contractions were actually the minor ones. My pregnancy went along very nicely and my husband stood by my side every moment. Having my husband by my side helped make the whole pregnancy a lot less stressful. I could not have asked for a better pregnancy. God was definitely by my side. I had no seizures while in labor. I had a C-section with an epidermal to comfort any pain I may have felt while giving birth to the baby.

On July 17, 1998, at 12:56 A.M., I had a healthy, beautiful baby boy, whom I named Michael Andrew Chillemi. He was born at 6 pounds 12 ounces. I still remember the loud cry he let out when I gave birth to him. The moment I saw my son, a healthy, beautiful baby that my husband and I had brought into this world, I knew then that nothing was impossible if you really set you heart on it.

He is now just about six months old at sixteen pounds and going strong. I never knew someone so small could eat so much! I have been enjoying motherhood and my epilepsy has not interfered with raising my son. Michael has been a tremendous joy to me and my husband.

I decided not to breast-feed instead I fed him with a formula called Neocate. I was always afraid to feed him my breast milk because I was not sure of how he would react to the Phenobarbital and Oxicarb. They say that Phenobarbital or Mysoline can make the babies sleepy or irritable. Women with epilepsy can breast-feed. It is a safe option because all medications are found in only small amounts of the breast milk. Yet because it is in the breast milk I choose to discard this option.

When I feel a seizure about to come, I put the baby down and give myself enough space to have the seizure. After the seizure, if I feel all right I go about my regular routine. If I am tired than I take a little nap with Michael. Epilepsy has not stopped me from having a beautiful baby and a wonderful family. I can be the best mother ever of epilepsy has not interfered with my life in any way shape of form. To survive and live happily, you need to think positively and have faith, faith in yourself.

SECTION FIVE

CLOSING THOUGHTS

Chapter 13

Journeying into the Millennium

As we journey into the year 2000 we look forward to what medical technology has in store for epileptics. Epilepsy is not being ignored. The medical world is constantly working on medicines and treatments for epilepsy. New medications for epilepsy are constantly becoming available. Diagnostic and surgical techniques are constantly being improved and new therapies for epilepsy are under research investigation. As we travel into the millennium new remedies lie ahead. There is promise for the millions who suffer with epilepsy.

In this year alone two medications were approved by the FDA for seizures. Lamictal (lamotrigine) a chewable dispersible tablet approved in June and Topamax approved in July.

Research alone has been active this year. Researchers from the university of Utah have discovered a genetic source of fever-induced childhood seizures by closely studying one family in Utah. This type of seizure is very similar to those seen in the general population, where approximately four of every 100 young children develop seizures when they run a high temperature.

Through a method called genetic linkage, the researchers were able to locate the chromosome associated with the seizures. They created a gene map, tracing who in the family inherited which chromosomes by following certain traits that they knew were located on a specific chromosome. They were even able to distinguish which section of the chromosome is involved. Researchers say the next step is to hone in on exactly which genes on the chromosomes are responsible for causing the convulsions.

Also, this year the American Academy of Neurology (AAN) Therapeutics and Technology Subcommittee approved the Vagus Nerve Stimulator (VNS). This was sais to bean effective and safe treatment for certain types of epilepsy. In 1997, the organization had termed the treatment "promising," but reserved its endorsement until further research could be conducted.

Since 1997, additional study has shown this treatment to be successful in many cases. The EO5 Study involved 254 people with epilepsy, ranging in ages of 13 to 60. All the patients had intractable partial seizures. After a three- to four-month observation period to establish the "normal" level of seizure activity for each participant, the VNS device was implanted. A few weeks later two groups were formed, with one receiving high stimulation and the other low stimulation for a period of three months.

Seizure frequency was reduced by an average of 28 percent in 94 subjects who had received high stimulation, while the low-stimulation group experienced an average 15 percent decline in the seizure frequency. This is roughly the same percentage that would improve if they used the newest seizure medications.

From all the data collected so far, the effectiveness of the treatment doesn't seem to wear off over time. In some cases, the participants continued to improve over time.

VNS involves surgically implanting an electrical device to stimulate the vagus nerve in the neck area. It's used to treat partial epilepsy in people when medication fails to provide improvement or causes adverse effects.

Though VNS is considered an effective treatment for epilepsy, the AAN still advises physicians to first evaluate each patient to determine if a surgical procedure could potentially cure the epilepsy.

Another research is also be done on a therapy called Magnetic Therapy. Transcranial magnetic stimulation (TMS) is a new field in neuroscience that uses powerful magnetic fields to alter brain activity. A number of preliminary studies have shown that TMS may be used to diagnose and/or treat a variety of clinical disorders. Best know for its use in treating depression, it also shows promise for helping anxiety disorders, schizophrenia, epilepsy, and movement disorders.

In TMS, an electromagnetic wire is placed on the scalp while a high intensity current is rapidly turned on and off. This creates a brief magnetic field that lasts about 100 to 200 microseconds. Due to the close physical proximity of the magnetic field to the brain, a flow of electrical current is induced into brain tissues. TMS is able to generate sufficient current such that electrical charges on the inside and outside of nerve cells become separated or depolarized. With present TMS technology, the depth of brain area that can be depolarized is two centimeters below the brain's surface.

Depolarization is also the desired goal of transcranial electric stimulation, more commonly called electroconvulsive therapy (ECT). During ECT, electrodes are placed on the scalp and direct electrical stimulation is applied. This produces a generalized seizure in the patient.

Unlike ECT, TMS can be applied with great precision to a particular area of the brain, and it does not stimulate pain receptors in the scalp. Generally patients are awake and alert during TMS therapy. Although earplugs are worn for safety, the procedure is performed on an outpatient basis and does not require anesthesia or analgesics. Most patients experience few side effects, except for occasional mild headache or discomfort at the stimulation site.

When placed over the brain's motor region, TMS elicits simple movements; over the visual region, the perception of light flashes. TMS does not cause memories, smells, or other complex psychological phenomenon. Repetitive and rapid TMS (rTMS) is used clinically, but can interfere with behavior and the processing of information when improperly administered.

While this new therapy is promising, the experts caution that more studies are needed before fully implementing TMS into the medical setting.

These are just a few of the researches that have been done this year. There are many studies that have been done and more that are being planned for the upcoming future. Some of the other studies include:

- Investigating neurochemical and cellular changes associated with seizures and the tendency toward having seizures
- Charting genes linked to epilepsy
- Studying changes in cellular metabolism during and after seizures
- Developing more effective drugs for epilepsy
- Creating and improving advanced techniques for mapping areas of the brain responsible for seizures (this will improve surgery for epilepsy)
- Developing and improving epileptic surgery
- Gaining a better understanding of seizures on children and adults
- The best is yet to come.

Appendix 1

FOODS, FATS AND THEIR CALORIES

NAME	SERVING	FAT	CALORIES
BREAD			
Bagel, Plain	1	2.0	200
French	1 Slice	1.0	100
Italian	1 Slice	0	85
Mixed Grain	1 Slice	1.0	65
Pita	1	1.0	165
Pumpernickel	1 Slice	1.0	80
Raisin	1 Slice	1.0	65
Rye (Light)	1 Slice	1.0	65
White (18 Slices per loaf)	1 Slice	1.0	65

NAME	SERVING	FAT	CALORIES
Whole-Wheat	1 Slice	1.0	70
Cereals			
Corn Flakes	1 cup	0	110
All-Bran	1 oz.	1.0	70
Bran Flakes Kellogg=s	1 oz.	1.0	90
Bran Flakes, Post	1 oz.	0.0	90
Cap=n Crunch	1 oz.	3.0	120
Fruit Loops	1 cup	0	110
Wheaties	1 cup	5	99
Cheerios	1 1/4	2	110
Raisin Bran Kellogg=s	1 oz.	1	90
Cream of Wheat	1 cup	0	100
Raisin Bran, Post	1 oz.	1.0	85
Wheat 1 Biscuit		0	80
Quaker Oatmeal	2/3	2	50
Quaker Puff Rice	1 cup	0	50
Frosted Flakes	1 oz.	0	110
Golden Grahams	1 oz.	1.0	110

NAME	SERVING	FAT	CALORIES
Grape- Nuts	1 oz.	0	100
Honey-Nut Cheerios	1 oz.	1.0	105
Rice Krispies	1 oz.	0	110
NAME	*SERVING*	*FAT*	*CALORIES*
Lucky Charms	1 oz.	1.0	110
Nature Valley Granola	1 oz.	5.0	125
Shredded Wheat	1 oz.	1	100
Product 19	1 oz.	0	110
Special K	1 oz.	0	110
Super Sugar Crisp	1 oz	0	105
Sugar Smacks	1 oz.	0	105
Total	1 oz.	1	100
Trix	1 oz.	0	110
Corn Flakes, Kellogg=s	1 oz.	0	110
NAME	*SERVING*	*FAT*	*CALORIES*
Cheeses			
Kraft American Singles	1 oz.	7.0	90

mozzarella/part skim	1 oz.	4.5	72
mozzarella/whole milk	1 oz.	7.0	90
Parmesan grated	1 table	1.5	23
hard	1 oz.	7.3	111
NAME	*SERVING*	*FAT*	*CALORIES*
Poultry			
w/skin roasted	2 breast	7.6	193
w/o skin roasted	2 breast	3.1	142
chicken leg		7.2	162
chicken thigh		9.2	180
Turkey			
grounded turkey		2	195
barbecued louis rich	3 2	5.0	135
oven roasted louis rich	3 2	3.0	115
dark meat w/skin roasted	3 2	11.5	221
w/out skin roasted	3 2	7.2	187

NAME	SERVING	FAT	CALORIES
Milk & Yogurt			
fat	2	3.0	115
frozen, non-fat	2	.2	81
fruit flavored			
low fat	1 cup	2.6	225
plain low			
fat	1 cup	3.5	144
NAME	SERVING	FAT	CALORIES
skim non-fat	1 cup	.4	127
whole milk	1 cup	7.4	139
2% milk	1 cup	.5	120
1% milk	1 cup	.3	100
NAME	SERVING	FAT	CALORIES
Pasta			
a noodle=s & rice			

regular	1 cup	.7	159
whole	1 cup	.6	159
wheat	1 cup	.6	183
Rice			
rice	1 cup		140
brown	2 cup	.6	116
long, grain & wild	2 cup	2.1	120
instant	1 cup	0	180
white	2 cup	1.2	111
spaghetti enriched	1 cup	1.0	159
NAME		**FAT**	**CALORIES**
Beef			
beef eyes of round		4.2	143
ground top ground		4.2	153
NAME	*SERVING*	*FAT*	*CALORIES*
beef tip round		5.9	157
beef top sirloin		6.1	165
beef top loin		8.0	176
beef tender loin		8.5	179

NAME		FAT	CALORIES
Ground Meat			
Ground Meat			
low fat ground beef		7	149
ground beef 85% lean		12	204
ground beef 80% lean		15	228
NAME		**FAT**	**CALORIES**
Seafood			
atlantic cod		1	89
lobster		1	83
salmon canned w/bone & liquid		5	118
smoked salmon		4	99
swordfish		4	158
tuna, canned in oil & drained		7	111
tuna, canned in water & drained		0	84
fried shrimp		10	206

NAME	SERVING	FAT	CALORIES
Vegetables			
artichoke boiled	1 med.	.2	53
black eyed peas	2 cup	.5	99
corn cream style		.4	93
frozen corn		.2	67
1 med.		2.6	105
frozen w/butter			
whole kernel		1.1	89
corn on the cob			
1 med.		.9	83
spinach	1 cup	0	10
broccoli	2 cup	11.5	189
carrot raw	1 med.	0	31
eggplant	1 cup	0	25
lettuce			
butterhead	1 head	0	20
crisphead	1 head	1	70
looseleaf	1 cup	0	10
peas	2 cup	0	67

NAME	SERVING	FAT	CALORIES
peppers, bell			
green	1	0	20
red	1	0	20
Potato=s/Beans/ Salad			
potato baked w/skin	1 med.	.2	220
french fries			
frozen	10 pieces	4.4	111
homemade		8.3	158
baked sweet	1 med	.1	118
potato salad	2 cup	11.5	189
soy beans	2 cup	7.7	149
caesar salad	1 cup	7.2	80
coleslaw	2 cup	14.2	147
NAME	SERVING	FAT	CALORIES
Fruits			
apples	1 med.	1	81
bananas		1	105
oranges		0	65

NAME	SERVING	FAT	CALORIES
raisins	1/3 cup	0	150
blueberries	1 cup	1	80
cantaloupe	2	1	95
cherries	10	1	50
grapefruit, white	2	0	40
grapes	10	0	35
lemons	1	0	15
NAME	SERVING	FAT	CALORIES
nectarines	1	1	65
peaches	1	0	35
pears			
D=Anjou	1	1	120
Bartlett	1	1	100
pineapple	1 cup	1	75
plums	1 large	0	35
raspberries	1 cup	1	60
strawberries	1 cup	1	45
NAME	SERVING	FAT	CALORIES
tangerines	1	0	35
watermelon	1 cup	1	50

fruit cocktail (heavy syrup)	2 cup	0	93

Epilepsy Clinical Research Centers and Organizations That Help Epilepsy

---

A.V. Delgado-Escueta, M.D.
West Los Angeles VA Medical Center
Wilshire and Sawtelle Blvds., Room 3405
Los Angeles, California 90073
(310) 824-4303 or 824-4448

Robert J Delorenzo, M.D., Ph.D.
Department of Neurology

Medical College of Virginia
Box 599, MCV Station

Richmond, Virginia 23298-0599
(804) 786-9720

Peter Kellaway, Ph.D
Baylor College of Medicine
1200 Moursund Avenue
Houston, Texas 77025
(713) 790-3109

R.H. Mattson, M.M.
Yale University School of
Medicine
333 Cedar Street
New Haven, Connecticut
06516
(203) 785-4086

William C. Dement, M.D.
Department of Psychiatry

and Behavioral Sciences
Building TD, Room 114

Stanford University School of Medicine
Standford, California 94305
(415) 723-8131

J.E. Engel, Jr, M.D., Ph.D.
University of Los Angeles

Department of Neurology, Room 1250
710 Westwood Plaza
Los Angeles, California 90024-1769
(310) 825-5745

James Ferrendelli, M.D.

Washington University School of Medicine
660 South Euclid Avenue
St. Louis, Missouri 63110

(314) 362-5262

Robert Gumnit, M.D.
MINCEP Epilepsy Care

5775 Wayzata Boulevard

J.O. McNamara, M.D.
Duke University School of
Medicine
P.O. Box 3005
Durham, North Carolina
27710
(919) 684-4241

G.A. Ojemann, M.D.
Duke University School of
Medicine
Seattle, Washington 98195
(206) 543-3573

W. Donald Shields, M.D.

UCLA School of Medicine
Department of Neurology
Los Angeles, California
90024-1769
(310) 825-6196

David A. Prince, M.D.
Standford   University
Medical Center
300 Pasteur Drive

Minneapolis, Minnesota 55416

(612) 525-2400

Richard A. Gillis, Ph.D
Georgetown University
3900 Reservoir Road, MN
Washington, DC 20007
(202) 687-8587

EPILEPSY FOUNDATION OF AMERICA
4351 Garden City Drive
*Land*over, MD 20785
(301) 459-3700

Epilepsy Foundation of New Jersey
Employment Department Suite 212
Trenton, NJ 08608
(609) 392-4900

National Epilepsy Library
1-800-EFA-4050

Epilepsy Information Service
Medical Center Boulevard
Winston-Salem, NC 27157-1078
1-800-642-0500

Standford, California
94305
(415) 723-6661

Internet Resources

www.efa.org
The Epilepsy Foundation is a national organization that works for people affected by seizures through research, education, advocacy and service. National programs include a toll-free informational service (1-800-EFA-1000), research, professional education, legal and legislative advocacy and employment issues.

Epilepsy Foundation of America Gene Discovery Project
www.epilepsygene.org
The purpose of this project is to educate families with epilepsy about current research in genetics and to join in a research partnership with international medical centers to identify the gene for epilepsy and their family.

American Academy of Neurology
www.aancom:80/home.html

American Academy of Pediatrics
www.aap.org

Child Neurology Society
www.umn.edu/cns

Child-Neuro Website
www.waisman.wisc.edu/child-neuro/

Free Electronic News From the AAMC

www.aamc.org/events/aamcstat/aamcnews.htm

International Bureau for Epilepsy
www.who.ch/programmes/ina/ngo-37.htm

International League against Epilepsy
www.websciences.org/engel
The international League against Epilepsy's objective is to advance and disseminate knowledge concerning epilepsy. Membership consists of national and professional organizations and individuals involved in research and interested in exchange of scientific information concerning epilepsy.

Epilepsy Ontario
www.epilepsyontario.org/links/index.html

AED (Antiepileptic Drug) Pregnancy Registry
1-888-233-2334
AED (antiepileptic Drug) Pregnancy Registry is the first North american Registry for pregnant women who are taking any AED-old or new, monotherapy or polytherapy to prevent seizures. All information is kept confidential. Educational materials will be provided. Enrolled women will be asked to provide through their doctors information about the health status of their infants. The findings will be analyzed to assess the fetal risk from all AED in pregnancy.

Registry Site Genetics & Teratology Unit
Massachusetts General Hospital
Fax: (617) 724-8307
Email: *aedregistry@helix.mgh.harvard.edu*
Web site: *http://neuro-www2.mgh.harvard.edu/aed/registry.nelk*

Appendix 3

GLOSSARY

Atonic Seizures (Also Called Drop Attacks)—A child or adult suddenly collapses and falls.

After 10 seconds to a minute he recovers, regains consciousness, and can stand and walk again.

Aura—An aura is a feeling that may warn the person who has it that a more severe seizure is about to begin. The aura is, in fact, the start of seizure activity in the brain before it spreads to other areas. Some people when experiencing an aura will develop a feeling of fear or sickness or an odd smell or taste. People who experience aura are warned ahead of time and are able to move away from hazards. Sometimes the more severe seizure does not follow, and all that happens is the sensation.

Complex Partial (Also known as Psychomotor or Temporal Lobe)—A complex partial seizure is known also as a psychomotor or temporal lobe seizure. This is a type of seizure in which the extra brain activity does not affect the whole brain. Although they call them "temporal lobe" seizures, they can occur in several areas of the brain. A complex partial seizure looks like a person is in a trance. The person goes through a series of movements over which they have no control. The movements vary from person to person.

A seizure of this type may start with a strange sensation such as, a feeling of fear, or a sudden sick feeling in the stomach, or even hearing or seeing something that isn't really there. The person stares blankly, and may make chewing movements with his mouth. He may move an arm, pull at clothing, get up and walk around all the time looking as if he's in a daze. Although not aware of things and people around him in the usual sense. A person having this seizure may follow simple directions if they are given a calm, friendly voice.

Some complex partial seizures produce more dramatic changes in behavior, including screaming, crying, moaning, laughing, disrobing, running, or apparent fear. There is no memory of what happened during the seizure period.

EFA—Epilepsy Foundation of America

Electroencephalogram (EEG)—An EEG is a machine that records the brain waves (electrical activity) picked up by tiny wires (electrodes) attached to various points on the patient scalp. The machine records electrical signals from the brain cells as wavy lines. The brain waves may show special patterns that may help the doctor decide whether the person has epilepsy. It also allows the doctor to identify what type of seizures the person is experiencing.

Encephalitis—An inflammation of the brain; usually caused by a virus

Epileptogenic—Causing epilepsy.

Epileptologist—A neurologist with special training in epilepsy.

Grand Mal Seizure (Also known as Generalized Tonic-clonic)—In this seizure, the whole brain is suddenly swamped with electrical energy. It often starts with a cry caused by air being suddenly forced out of the lungs. The person falls to the ground and becomes unconscious. The individual's body will stiffen briefly and then they begin having jerking movements. Biting their tongue during this episode is common for the individual. Bubbling saliva may also appear around the person's mouth. Their breathing also may get very shallow and even stop for a few moments, causing the skin to turn a bluish color. Jerking movements then begin to slow and the seizures will end naturally. The bladder and bowel control is sometimes lost. When consciousness returns to the person, they may feel confused and sleepy. An individual may even experience some memory loss. Occasionally they require only a very short recovery period, and most people can go back to their normal activities after awhile. If the seizure is prolonged then medical attention is critical.

Infantile Spasms—These are clusters of quick, sudden movements that start between 3 months and two years. If a child is sitting up, the head will fall forward, and the arms will flex forward. If lying down, the knees will be drawn up, with the arms and head flexed forward as if the baby is reaching for support.

MRI—Provides a three-dimensional picture for identifying damaged areas of the brain.

Myoclonic Jerk—Brief muscle jerk; may involve muscles on one or both sides of the body; may be normal (example, as one falls asleep) or caused by a seizure or other disorders.

Myoclonic Seizures—A brief muscle jerk resulting from an abnormal discharge of brain electrical activity; usually involves muscles on both sides of the body, most often the shoulders or upper arms.

Petit Mal Seizure (Also Known as Absence or Focal Seizure)—They look like daydreaming, or blank staring ending abruptly, lasting only a few seconds, most common in children. May be accompanied by rapid blinking, some chewing movements of the mouth. Child or adult is unaware of what's going on during the seizure, but quickly returns to full awareness once it has stopped. May result in learning difficulties if not recognized and treated. These seizures happen so quickly that others around that person may not even notice the seizure occurring.

Positron Emission Tomography (PET)—A diagnostic test that uses a low and safe dose of radioactive compound to measure metabolic activity in the brain; can identify areas of decreased metabolism corresponding to the area from which the seizure arise; helping in planning epileptic surgery.

Reflex Epilepsies—Seizure caused by certain conditions or stimuli, such as flashing lights or jazz music.

Single-photon Emission Computed Tomography (SPET)- A diagnostic test that uses a low and safe dose of radioactive compound to measure blood flow in the brain; not as sensitive as the PET.

Simple Partial—Jerking may begin in one area of body, arm, leg, or face. Can't be stopped, but patient stays awake and aware. Jerking may proceed from one area of the body to another, and sometimes spreads to become a convulsive seizure.

Partial sensory seizures may not be obvious to an onlooker. Patient experiences a distorted environment. May see or hear things that aren't there, may feel unexplained fear, sadness, anger, or joy. May have nausea, experience odd smells, and have a generally "funny" feeling in the stomach.

Spell—A period, bout, or episode of illness or indisposition; refers to seizures or other disorders that produce brief episodes of behavioral change.

Status Epilepticus—A prolonged seizure (usually longer than 30 minutes) or series of repeated seizures; a continuous state of seizure activity; may occur in almost any seizure type.

Video-EEG Monitoring—A technique for recording the behavior and the EEG of a patient simultaneously; changes in behavior can be correlated with changes in the EEG; useful for making the diagnosis of epilepsy and localizing the seizure focus.

Generic Name	Brand Name	Indications
Acettazolamide	Diamox	Myoclonic seizures
Adrenocorticotropic	Cortrosyn	Infantile spasms
Carbazazepine	Tegretol	Partial seizures, tonic-clonic seizures
Clonazepam	Klonopin	Myoclonic Seizures, absence seizures
Clorazepate	Tranxene	Absence seizures, partial seizures
Ethosuxmide	Zarontin	Myoclonic Seizures, absence seizures
Felbamate	Felbatol	Partial seizures, tonic-clonic seizures, atonic seizures, tonic seizures
Gabapentin	Neurontin	Partial seizures, tonic-clonic seizures
Lamotrigine	Lamictal	Partial seizures, tonic-clonic seizures
Lorazepam	Ativan	Status epilepticus, seizure clusters
Mephopbarbital	Mebaral	Partial seizures, tonic-clonic seizures, myoclonic Seizures
Phenobarbital	Luminal (and others)	Partial seizures, tonic-clonic seizures
Phenytoin	Dilantin	Partial seizures, tonic-clonic seizures
Prednisone	——	Infantile spasms
Primidone	Mysoline	Partial seizures, tonic-clonic seizures
Trimethadione	Tridione	Absence seizures
Valproare	Depakene Depakote	Absence seizures tonic-clonic seizures, myoclonic Seizures, partial seizures

BIBLIOGRAPHY

A Guide to understanding and Living with Epilepsy, Orrin Devinsky, Philadelphia: F.A. Davis Company, 1994

Stop the Insanity!, Susan Powters. New York 1993
Simon & Schuster,

Yoga For Health, Richard Elittlemano. Canada: Ballantine Books, a division of Random House, Inc., in New York, 1983

Epilepsy Foundation of America. Trenton, New Jersey, 1995

Maryland & also the division in Prescription for Nutritional Healing, James F. Balch, MD Phyllis A. Baich C.N.C., Avery Publishing Group Inc., Garden City Park, New York
1990

Booklet written by Epilepsy Foundation of America. Questions and Answers About seizure disorders. Publication of this material is made possible by a grant from Parke-Davis. Division of Warner-Lambert Company. Opinions are those of the author and may not necessarily reflect the views of the sponsor. What causes a person to develop epilepsy? (1983);4:1 What kinds of seizures do people with epilepsy have? (1983) Some seizures look like sleepwalking. Complex partial seizures. (1983);3:3-4 Most seizures don't injure the brain. What is an aura? (1983);1:5

Sometimes surgery can stop seizures. When is epilepsy treated by surgery? (1983);3:10-11
Q & A about treatment. When kinds of tests are used in evaluation of a person who may have epilepsy? (1983);1:9 How many people in the U.S. have epilepsy? (1983); 3: 1
Sometimes surgery can stop seizures. How many people in the U.S. have epilepsy? (1983); 3: 1

Dr. Michael Chillemi D.C.. Abstract of Epilepsy. 1997
Q & A about treatment. When kinds of tests are used in evaluation of a person who may have epilepsy? 1983;1:9 What is epilepsy? 1983; 1: 1

Staying In Touch. Schuler, Sadowski & Bloodgood, Inc. Pregnancy Epilepsy. 1997; 8:1

"Surgery techniques offers hope" The Detroit News 11th May 1992 pg. 1E. Preoperative test span wide range, "Surgery for Epilepsy"Epilepsy Foundation of America,

Epilepsy USA vol. 29, Sept. 1996.

Sperling, Michael R. "temporal lobectomy for refractory epilepsy", The Journal of the American Medical Association, vol.276 pg.470, 14th Aug. 1996.

Sternberg, Steve "Controversial surgery benefits epileptics. (Anterior temporal lobectomy)", Science News, vol.150, pg102, 17th Aug. 1996.

America Online. Attitude and Healing. By Richard "Medicine Bear" Cantrell. 1998

Rose Medical Center. How To Fight & Conquer Stress. 1993

America Epilepsy Society. Health ResponseAbility Systems, Inc. 1997;1:3-5

America Epilepsy Society. Peter Hauri PhD and Shirly Linde, PhD. No More Sleepless Nights.1997;1

Segal, Julia, Phantasy in Everyday Life (1985); Watkins, May, Walking Dreams, 3d ed. (1984).
Epilepsy Foundation of America. Questions and Answers about Epilepsy. What is epilepsy?
1983; 1: 1

Jacqueline French MD. The Long-term Therapeutic Management of Epilepsy. Ann Intern Med.1994;120:411- 422.

Staying In Touch. Schuler, Sadowski & Bloodgood, Inc. Pregnancy Epilepsy. 1997;8:1 8."

Surgery techniques offers hope" The Detroit News 11th May 1992 pg. 1E.

Preoperative test span wide range, "Surgery for Epilepsy"Epilepsy Foundation of America, Epilepsy USA vol. 29, Sept. 1996.

Sperling, Michael R. "temporal lobectomy for refractory epilepsy", The Journal of the American Medical Association, vol.276 pg.470, 14th Aug. 1996.

Sternberg, Steve "Controversial surgery benefits epileptics. (Anterior temporal lobectomy)", Science News, vol.150, pg102, 17th Aug. 1996.

Connections. Schuler, Sadowski & Bloodgood, Inc. Guess Who Had Epilepsy. 1993

Epilepsy Foundation of America, Inc., Landover, MD. Glaxo Wellcome, Inc. Pregnancy and the Developing Child. 1997

Epilepsy Foundation of America, Inc., Landover, MD. Glaxo Wellcome, Inc. Pregnancy and the mother's Health.1997
Epilepsy Foundation of America, Inc., Landover, MD. Glaxo Wellcome, Inc. Parenting concerns for the mother with epilepsy.1997

Grolier, Inc. Exercise.1997 Bibliography: Fentem, P. H., et al., Benefits of Exercise (1990); Froelichek, V. F., Exercise Testing and Training (1983); Miller, D. K., and Allen, T. E., Fitness, 4th ed. (1990); Smith, E. L., and Serfass, R. C., eds., Exercise and Aging (1981); Strauss, R. H., Sports Medicine (1984).

Grolier, Inc. Human Nutrition.1997 Bibliography: Barnard, Neal, Food for Life (1993); Bourne, G. H., ed., International Nutrition in Health and Disease (1987); Burton, B. T., and Foster, W. R., Human Nutrition, 4th ed. (1988); Carper, J., Food, Your Miracle Medicine (1993); Clayman, C. B., Diet and Nutrition (1991); Guthrie, H. A., and Picciano, M. F., Human Nutrition (1994); Hamilton, E. M., et al., Nutrition, 5th ed. (1991); Klurfeld, D. M., ed., Human Nutrition, 8 vols. (1993); Lapp, F. M., Diet for a Small Planet, 20th ed. (1991); Sax, R., The Way We Eat (1994); Sims, C., and Roderick, G., Introductory Food Science (1995); Wolff, C. B., Nutrition and Fitness, 2d ed. (1995).;

Groiler, Inc. Yoga.1997

Grolier, Inc. The Psychology of Fantasy. 1997 Bibliography: Klinger, Eric, Daydreaming (1990);

Epilepsy Foundation of America. In Touch.1997

Holistic Herbal (1996) David Hoffmann; Black Cohosh, Relaxation Exercises.

Jacqueline French MD. The Long-term Therapeutic Management of Epilepsy. Ann Intern Med.1994;120:411- 422.

Dr. Michael Chillemi D.C.. Abstract of Epilepsy. 1997

America Online. Attitude and Healing. By Richard "Medicine Bear" Cantrell.1998

Rose Medical Center. How To Fight & Conquer Stress. 1993

America Online. Attitude and Healing. By Richard "Medicine Bear" Cantrell. 1998

America Epilepsy Society. Health ResponseAbility Systems, Inc. 1997;1:3-5.

America Epilepsy Society. Peter Hauri PhD and Shirly Linde, PhD. No More Sleepless Nights. 1997;1

Fever- Induced Seizures in Children Can Have Long-term Effects. Mediconsult.com 1999

Magnetic Therapy: New Kid on the Block in Neuropsychiatry. Mediconsult.com 1999

Researchers Get to the Core of Childhood Seizures. Medoconsult.com 1999

Nerve Stimulation Device Effective in Stopping Seizure Activity. Mediconsult.com 1999

ABOUT THE AUTHOR

Stacey Chillemi, is college graduate from Richard Stockton College in Pomona New Jersey with a Bachelor of Arts, in Marketing. She's received awards in her achievements and certificates in recognition for her outstanding efforts in trying to improve society. She has been an active participant in organizations and activities. She has been a role model to many individuals. She has written many articles on epilepsy, such as *How Exercise Can Help Your Seizures, Coping with Epilepsy, Can Women With Epilepsy Have Babies and Why Children Have Seizures.* She has also written self-help articles, such as *10 Steps to Self-confidence, Seven Steps to Loving Yourself, 4 Steps to High Self-esteem and Greatest relief for stress*: Take some time each day for yourself. She appeared twice on News 12 on the talk show New Jersey Women and has had articles written about her efforts to help people with epilepsy. Stacey Chillemi, contributes her time in helping people with epilepsy and making society more aware of the disorder. Stacey lives in New Jersey with her husband and two children. If you would like to contact her you can e-mail her at epilepsyusa@aol.com